365 SKINNY SMOOTHIES

DELICIOUS RECIPES TO HELP YOU GET SLIM AND STAY HEALTHY EVERY DAY OF THE YEAR

DANIELLA CHACE, MSc, CN

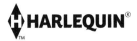

365 SKINNY SMOOTHIES

ISBN-13: 978-0-373-89299-0

The health advice presented in this book is intended only as an informative resource guide to help you make informed decisions; it is not meant to replace the advice of a physician or to serve as a guide to self-treatment. Always seek competent medical help for any health condition or if there is any question about the appropriateness of a procedure or health recommendation.

Library of Congress Cataloging-in-Publication Data
Chace, Daniella.

  365 skinny smoothies : delicious recipes to help you get slim and stay healthy every day of the year / Daniella Chace.

    pages cm
    Includes bibliographical references and index.

ISBN 978-0-373-89299-0 (paperback)
1. Smoothies (Beverages) 2. Diet therapy. 3. Weight loss.
I. Title. II. Title: Three hundred sixty-five skinny smoothies.
  TX815.C43 2014
  641.2'6--dc23

           2013046005

www.Harlequin.com
Printed in U.S.A.

CONTENTS

INTRODUCTION

Recipes for a Skinny Life

The smoothie recipes in *365 Skinny Smoothies* are nutritious elixirs designed to promote weight loss and increase energy. As a nutritionist, I know that smoothies are a dream come true because they can be a vehicle for macronutrients such as protein, essential fatty acids (EFAs) and complex carbohydrates, as well as micronutrients such as vitamins, minerals and phytonutrients.

I started making smoothies 20 years ago when I worked with cancer patients who needed concentrated amounts of protein and nutrients to support their immune systems throughout their healing process. I found that nutrient-dense foods and supplements could be added to delicious concoctions to create powerful healing drinks that taste delicious.

I use peer-reviewed studies and carefully choose the research I use when creating recipes for specific health outcomes. Therefore, while creating the weight-loss smoothies in *365 Skinny Smoothies,* I culled through hundreds of food-nutrient studies to find the most effective foods for increasing muscle and decreasing body fat. The medicinal smoothie recipes in this book will help you lose weight in various ways, such as reducing body fat storage by decreasing insulin stimulation, reducing cellulite by triggering the release of stored water (edema) and increasing enzymes that will help shed body fat.

A quick search for weight-loss smoothies online will turn up a plethora of misinformation as well as high-calorie, sugar-laden recipes created by smoothie enthusiasts who may not know much about nutrition. However, the studies referenced here and the nutrition tips are all based on empirical evidence. When you incorporate these smoothies into your daily routine, along with exercise and a healthy diet, these recipes can have a profound and direct effect on your health and your weight.

YOUR KITCHEN AS A LEARNING LAB

By trying out the recipes in this book, you are essentially creating a lab in your kitchen by experimenting with various nutrients that boost weight loss. Each recipe introduces a weight-loss concept, such as adding probiotic supplements and cultured foods; increasing phytochemicals found in greens and berries; increasing spices that reduce inflammation; hydrating with electrolytes; stocking up on frozen berries and dry goods; and adding protein such as hemp, chia or protein supplement powders to your smoothies.

You'll quickly master the basics of smoothie making, and you'll soon be ready to start customizing your own smoothies based on your taste preferences and nutrient needs. For example, my favorite morning combination is coconut water, banana, nonfat Greek yogurt, wild blueberries, protein powder and probiotics powder (see the January 30 recipe, "Chace's Morning Boost" in Chapter 4). However, everyone's tastes and needs vary, so you may prefer, for instance, cherry juice for the base and you may need more vitamin C. Thus, you might choose to add citrus and greens to your breakfast smoothie recipe.

HOW TO USE THIS BOOK

The recipe chapters are organized by perishable ingredients—this means that each month's recipes are grouped together according to their staple ingredient in order to ease your shopping burden. This allows you to use up the fresh foods that you've purchased so there is less waste, and you won't have to fill your refrigerator with too many new products all at once. If you follow the book from beginning to end, you will be buying the minimal amount of new foods each week.

In addition, seasonal ingredients are the focus for each month, which makes it easier to find ingredients that aren't available year-round. Keep in mind that you can always alter a recipe if you can't find a particular ingredient, so it's not necessary for you to hunt down anything unusual or hard to find in your area. I've provided ideas for alternates to use when you're out of a particular ingredient in the ingredient list provided in Chapter 2 (see page 11).

Rest assured that the recipes in this book are all low calorie. The ones that have fewer than 250 calories are considered to be snacks—little pick-me-ups to drink between meals or as an addition to a light meal. You can enjoy these smoothies several times throughout the day without racking up the calories. There are a few smoothies that contain more than 250 calories, and these can be used as meal replacements.

With each recipe you'll find the amount of calories, fat, carbohydrates, fiber and protein for each smoothie. The goal in creating a balanced smoothie is to keep the calories and fat content low (unless the fat is from a healthy source such as avocado) and to have as much fiber and protein as possible. The nutritional content breakdowns are listed per serving. Some of the recipes are just one serving while some are larger and make two servings. Recipes can be doubled easily or divided in half to meet your needs depending on whether you're making smoothies for one or two people.

In the old days we had milkshakes and slushy-type drinks with lots of fat, sugar, calories and food coloring. Now we know that we can make nutritious smoothies that have a "comfort food" texture and flavor without all of the unhealthy ingredients. To this end, these smoothies are not only full of weight-loss nutrients but also are delicious and rich with satisfying flavor.

Each smoothie is composed of a balance of protein and fiber to allow for a slow release of the carbohydrates, which gives your body time to burn the calories as energy rather than storing them as fat in the thighs or abdominal region. The recipes also contain essential fatty acids that increase the enzymes that help us release the body fat we already have so we can burn it for energy as well. Many of these recipes contain natural fiber from their fruits, vegetables, seeds and nuts; however, adding a half teaspoon of a fiber supplement to each smoothie will further reduce the glycemic load of the smoothie, which means you'll get an even longer energy boost. All you really need to get started is a blender, a liquid (which can be as simple as water), fresh or frozen produce (such as a banana) and some protein (nuts, seeds, protein powder). Toss them in your blender or food processor, blend until smooth and drink right away.

A YEAR OF EXPLORING SMOOTHIES

Keep in mind that everyone's taste buds are different. Some prefer hot and spicy, some prefer sour, and others prefer sweet and creamy. This book has something for everyone. My intention is to introduce you to several new flavors and combinations each month so that you can try them until you find your favorites.

In the following chapter I have illuminated some fascinating and little-known nutrition secrets. I reveal tips that I share with clients to help them lose weight. As you work your way through the recipes in this book you will be incorporating these strategies and learning from experience which ones work best for you.

I hope you enjoy sampling the flavors of life while you energize your body one smoothie at a time!

CHAPTER 1

Nutrition Secrets for Losing Weight with Smoothies

This chapter offers some secrets that can help you get your metabolism burning at peak rate. We each have different and specific nutritional needs. For example, at any given point in time we may have nutrient deficiencies, or our metabolism may be effected by toxins or our immune systems may be triggered by food allergens. You can test your metabolism by experimenting with the following strategies to see what works for you. For example, reducing exposure to toxins will help some people shed pounds immediately, while others see more weight loss when they avoid foods they're allergic to. You'll know you're impacting your ability to lose weight when you start to shed pounds.

MINIMIZE SUGAR

Simple sugar is unhealthy because it delivers empty calories (calories without nutrients), and raises cholesterol and triglyceride levels, causing insulin resistance, inflammation and insulin fluctuations that can lead to weight gain. To monitor your intake of sugar, check the sugar content on food labels. Keep in mind that sugars are simple carbohydrates and are included in the total number of carbohydrates listed on a label.

Our daily recommended carbohydrate intake, which includes fruits and vegetables, is calculated based on our size and activity level. The American Diabetes Association recommends about 45–60 grams of carbohydrate at a meal. All of the smoothies in this book provide the number of grams of carbs per serving. This carb number includes both complex carbohydrates, such as those from whole fruits, as well as sugars from fruit juices. My recipes contain between 15 and 30 carbs per smoothie, which is clearly well under the ADA's recommended intake. I have carefully designed the smoothies in this book to be low carb and low calorie.

ADD PROTEIN TO SMOOTHIES TO INCREASE MUSCLE AND DECREASE FAT

Adding protein to smoothies supplies the amino acids we need for efficient weight loss. Studies show that protein reduces the appetite as well as food cravings, and it also provides the amino acids that drive metabolism. The amount of protein we need varies depending on our activity level, age and gender but to give you a general idea, most adults need about 50 grams of dietary protein daily. To learn more check out the Centers for Disease Control (cdc.gov), which provides a Recommended Dietary Allowance for Protein chart on their website.

The following chart provides some examples of my favorite sources of protein for smoothies.

Protein powders	14-32 grams in 3 tablespoons
Greek yogurt	16-20 grams in ½ cup
Cottage cheese	14 grams in ½ cup
Yogurt	10 grams in ½ cup
Hulled hemp seed	5-7 grams in 2 tablespoons
Chia seed	6 grams in 2 tablespoons
Hemp protein powder	5 grams in 2 tablespoons
Nuts	5 grams in ¼ cup

DRINK PROTEIN WITH YOUR CARBS

The ideal weight loss smoothie is low calorie and protein-enhanced to supply just enough fuel for consistent energy without the fat storage. Protein is a key macronutrient for weight loss, as it supplies amino acids that are the building blocks for many of the biological functions in our bodies. Increasing the protein in our diets helps provide the nutrients we need to keep our metabolism at peak performance. Protein foods, such as chia seed, hulled hemp seed and protein powders, can be added to smoothies to help balance the carbohydrates. Protein and fat help to slow the breakdown (digestion) of the entire meal, thus reducing the amount of sugar from the carbohydrate being released into the bloodstream at one time. Therefore, the protein helps give our metabolic processes time to use the calories from our food as energy rather than storing the calories as body fat.

AVOID TOXINS TO LOSE WEIGHT MORE QUICKLY!

Some toxins have a direct link to obesity, because they affect the liver. When the liver is busy cleaning up toxins, it can't properly break down insulin, which continues to circulate longer in your bloodstream, grabbing up sugar and storing it away as fat. The more toxins, the more body fat storage!

GLASS IS HEALTHIER THAN PLASTIC

Avoid phthalates, such as bisphenol A (BPA), which are toxins found in most plastics. Studies have found that exposure to these compounds through our food and water may be a causative factor in the development of obesity. You can minimize your exposure to these compounds by purchasing and storing foods and juices in glass rather than plastic. Foods and juices are increasingly available in glass containers, as many food product manufacturers are becoming aware of consumers' health concerns around the toxicity of plastics.

BUY ORGANIC WHEN IT MATTERS

Avoid agricultural chemicals by buying organic products. The Environmental Working Group (EWG.org) has a handy list of the "Dirty Dozen," which are the most heavily sprayed types of produce. For example, apples, celery, cherry tomatoes, cucumbers, grapes, hot peppers, nectarines, peaches, spinach and strawberries are all heavily sprayed, so it's best to buy organic. The USDA's "Organic" seal also lets you know a product is free of genetically modified organisms (GMOs), which is important because GMOs are inherently grown with the use of more agricultural chemicals than other types of crops. The EWG also provides a "Clean Fifteen" list, which is the least sprayed types of produce such as avocado, cantaloupe, grapefruit, kiwi, mango, papaya and pineapple. It's not as important to buy organic when it comes to these foods.

SWEETEN WITH FIBER

Sometimes we want to add a little sweetness to a smoothie. This can be done with fiber-rich foods such as dates, prunes and figs. They add sweet flavor but they break down slowly in our bodies because of their fiber. This is a huge benefit because slowing the digestion of the carbohydrates gives our bodies longer lasting energy and less storage of body fat.

BE A FOOD DETECTIVE: READ NUTRITION LABELS

When you buy food products such as yogurt, be sure to read the "Nutrition Facts" labels to see how much sugar, fat and protein is in each serving. Some yogurts have as much sugar as a candy bar. And don't assume that less sugar equals low calorie. Often, sugar-free or reduced-sugar foods have even more calories than their original counterparts and may contain harmful artificial sweeteners.

Nutrition facts food labels are on most food products and make it possible to calculate the macronutrient (carbohydrates, protein and fat) levels in each serving of that food or drink. It's important to be aware that the numbers listed reflect one serving. Always take a quick glance at the number of servings per container even when it seems like it should be obvious. For example, small bottles of juice that most of us would intend to drink as one serving are often designated as 2 or even 3 servings. This is common with food labeling. You can avoid this trap by simply being aware and looking at the number of servings and then multiplying the number of grams of carbs by the servings number to get the total number of carbs for that product.

AVOID INFLAMMATION TRIGGERS AND LOSE WATER WEIGHT

Inflammation is becoming a common health issue, as so many people suffer from food allergies and toxicities due to food processing and sugar content. Inflammation can cause bloating, joint pain, headaches, stiff back and cellulite. However, by reducing the body's inflammation, cellulite seems to magically disappear as we excrete extra water weight.

Therefore, avoid food allergens that cause inflammation. Some of the most common allergenic foods are wheat and gluten, corn, eggs, refined sugar, milk and soy. Many people who react to dairy foods can still digest yogurt, however. Yogurt is a cultured product, which means it contains probiotic organisms that help break down the natural sugars—the lactose—making it easier to digest and assimilate. In my nutrition practice, my clients have reported losing up to 15 pounds of water weight within days of removing an allergenic food from the diet. Keep this in mind as some of your "body fat" may just be water weight from inflammation.

NUTRIENTS BOOST METABOLISM

We use nutrients in our bodies 24/7. If we develop nutrient deficiencies, this can slow our metabolism down and even halt some systems. For example, protein, glutathione, zinc, chromium and B vitamins are all critical nutrients in metabolism. A high-quality daily supplement, such as MediClear powder from Thorne Research, can be added to smoothies and will replenish nutrients daily. Berries and other superfoods such as pomegranate, cinnamon and holy basil are so rich in nutrients that they're like an antioxidant supplement themselves, especially when eaten daily.

DRINK YOUR SMOOTHIE IMMEDIATELY AFTER BLENDING

Smoothies do not travel well. The ingredients start to separate and oxidize almost immediately after blending. Try to drink your smoothies within a few minutes after blending while the nutrients are still fresh and vital.

A SMOOTHIE A DAY IS THE SKINNY WAY

Studies on the weight-loss effects of different food nutrients are continuously being reported. The research is very exciting, but keep in mind that the results are based on daily exposure to those nutrients. For example, we can't expect fiber or turmeric to help us lose weight if we ingest them only once a week. However, when we incorporate these nutrients into our daily routine, they can have a profound effect on our health. Our bodies are in a constant process of cell turnover, hormone production, and fat gain and release. By incorporating certain nutrients into our daily smoothies we support our bodies in the continual process of fat loss and muscle gain.

PROBIOTICS ARE KEY TO DIGESTION AND WEIGHT LOSS

There are thousands of different healthy bacteria that live in our gut, orchestrating our metabolic functions. Without proper gut flora we can't absorb nutrients such as polyphenols. Keep this in mind as you read about the powerful phytochemical nutrient studies throughout the book. We need a healthy gut flora for proper digestion and nutrient metabolism. We get these important organisms via cultured products such as cultured coconut milk, yogurt, kefir and supplements.

A "SMOOTHIE SNACK" VS. A "SMOOTHIE MEAL"

As mentioned in the Introduction, smoothies that are low in calories (fewer than 250 calories) are perfect little energizers between meals. Energy-dense smoothies with more than 250 calories can be used as meal replacements. Keep in mind that a 250 to 350 calorie smoothie is still fairly low in calories, and you may need to supplement it with a snack if you are active or have a higher calorie need. Most of the smoothies in this book are low-calorie energizers.

EFAs HELP BURN BODY FAT

We need essential fatty acids (EFAs)—which are healthful fats from foods such as avocado, nuts and seeds—for our skin and cells, nerves and fat-burning enzymes. EFAs are the essential oils/fats that we need to take in through our diet, as we can't produce these internally. Just one gram of EFAs per day appears to increase the production of fat-burning enzymes. One gram of EFAs is about 1 teaspoon of chia seed or 2 teaspoons of hulled hemp seed. In the recipes that follow, I generally recommend adding 1–2 tablespoons of chia seed, hulled hemp seed or protein powder to each smoothie to boost protein as well as EFAs.

ADDING FIBER TO SMOOTHIES IS KEY TO BLOOD SUGAR CONTROL

When we make smoothies, we're blending rather than juicing so that we retain the fiber from the fruits and vegetables we're including. This is beneficial because essential minerals attach themselves to this fiber. Also fiber holds onto water as it moves through the digestive tract, helping us hydrate. This allows the body to absorb water as needed, which vastly improves hydration (see the discussion about the importance of hydration that follows). Additionally, when fiber is added to a smoothie it helps reduce the glycemic load of the entire drink. The glycemic load is a system that assigns a number to specific foods based on how much they will increase a person's blood sugar level when eaten. For example, oranges are low at 40 while sugar is high at 100. When we add fiber to our meals we can reduce the overall glycemic load of that meal, as fiber slows the breakdown of foods in the digestive tract. This slows the release of its nutrients into the bloodstream. Thus reducing the risk for a spike in blood sugar, which triggers the pancreas to respond with insulin. Once insulin has been released into the bloodstream, its job is to shunt the sugar into cells for energy and the excess is stored away as fat. Therefore, increasing fiber in our meals and smoothies helps reduce the insulin response, which helps reduce the potential for calories to be stored away as body fat. There are many high-quality fiber products on the market these days—such as glucoman-nan, pectin, chicory fiber and acacia fiber—that are gentle and dissolve well in smoothies.

SMOOTHIES ENHANCE HYDRATION

Dehydration may give us the false signal that we are hungry when actually we are simply thirsty and in need of water and possibly electrolytes. Coconut water, fruit juices, and fruits and vegetables will boost water content and electrolytes in smoothies. You can also stay hydrated by drinking filtered water throughout the day and adding ice to your smoothies. Ice also helps emulsify (blend together) the smoothie. Adding liquids to smoothies, such as green tea, herbal teas and coconut water, can also increase hydration.

BREAKFAST KICK-STARTS YOUR METABOLISM

Once you leave the house, the day can get pretty busy. You might eat out or forget to take supplements. Having a daily morning smoothie is an effective weight-loss strategy. By get-ting that morning boost of nutrients and protein, you'll be starting the day off right no matter where the day takes you. Eating breakfast, especially a high-protein breakfast, also helps those who have lost weight keep it off. Studies have found that people who miss their morning meal are more likely to be obese.

INCREASE SPICES AND HERBS
BUT DECREASE SUGAR, FAT AND SALT

Holy basil, turmeric powder and black pepper provide pow-erful nutrients for weight loss. The world's oldest medical system, the Ayurvedic Medicine system of India, uses culi-nary herbs daily for the prevention and treatment of disease and imbalance. In India they use turmeric and black pepper to reduce inflammation, and they use holy basil (Tulsi) to balance blood sugar. Holy basil is a medicinally potent herb that has an amazing fragrance and flavor and happens to be a perfect smoothie ingredient. Studies have found that its antioxidants have a positive effect on blood sugar levels. It also contains active compounds, such as ursolic acid, rosmarinic acid, carvacrol and linalool, that each provide powerful health benefits. Ursolic acid has been found to inhibit certain cancer cell types; rosmarinic acid has antianxiety effects; carvacrol reduces inflammation; and the scent of linalool has been found to reduce stress. Whenever I'm watering my holy basil plants I breath the fragrance in and feel relaxed and happy.

Unfortunately we don't use many culinary herbs in the United States. In fact, the standard American diet relies heavily on sugar, fat and salt for flavor. By adding spices and herbs to foods we create flavor, move away from sugar, fat and salt, and also add nutrients that help us lose weight and keep us healthy.

You now have the power and knowledge to experiment and start your weight-loss journey!

CHAPTER 2

The Essential Weight-Loss Smoothie Ingredients

One of the key rules for weight loss is to take in (eat and drink) only as many calories as you can burn so that your body doesn't store the extra calories away as body fat. Store-bought and restaurant smoothies can be super-sized and, besides adding unwanted calories and other harmful ingredients, they are generally made of processed foods that are void of nutritional value. A quick scan of these products online shows us that they often contain a whopping 700 calories or more. Buying packaged or pre-made smoothies can get expensive and downright cost prohibitive for many. Making them at home gives you more control over the expense, the flavors and the quality of the ingredients. In this chapter, I have included a list of essential ingredients for making healthy smoothies at home. Many of these smoothie ingredients have a long shelf life, or they are frozen ingredients that will last for months in the freezer, which makes it easy to stock up. A few ingredients will need to be purchased fresh as they have a shorter shelf life. In either case, this is noted in the preparation and storage section, which is after each ingredient. You may want to start with the recipe section of this book and make your grocery list according to the recipes laid out for that week. The recipes are clustered by their most perishable ingredient, which will minimize the number of trips to the grocery store.

I've included tips on their nutritional value and how these nutrients improve our health and support weight loss. Feel free to alter the recipes to remove ones that you don't like and to add in the ingredients you like most. Enjoy!

ALMOND MILK

Almond milk is a beverage made from ground almonds and provides an alternative to dairy milk for vegans and those allergic to dairy. It's slightly sweet, provides protein and has a low calorie count with only about 40 calories per cup, which is less than a third of the calories of many of the milk alternatives, such as rice milk.

Preparation and storage: Almond milk comes premade and is usually housed in a Tetra Pak (aseptic package), so it does not need to be refrigerated until opened, and it has a long shelf life. It is available in several flavors and varieties, including plain, vanilla, low-fat or full-fat versions. Fresh, homemade almond milk is absolutely delicious in smoothies, in tea or coffee, over oatmeal or just as a cold milk drink alternative. To make your own almond milk, soak 1 cup of almonds in water overnight, then drain and rinse. Combine the soaked almonds in a blender with 2 cups of water and blend well. Strain it through cheesecloth to remove the almond meal and collect the fresh, sweet, nutty almond milk. Fresh almond milk lasts for about 2 days when refrigerated.

ALMONDS

Almonds are a rich source of vitamin E, protein, fiber, B vitamins, minerals and healthful fats. They also provide phytosterols, which help lower cholesterol levels. Whole almonds, almond butter and my favorite, roasted and chopped almonds, are often sold in bulk and are available at food co-ops, as they're used to make roasted almond butter. They are also available online. All forms of almonds can be used in smoothies. If you don't have almonds, alternative ingredients include cashews, hazelnuts, pecans and pistachios.

Preparation and storage: Roasted almonds are available pre-chopped, so they blend well. If you have a low-power blender, you may need to chop your nuts a bit before tossing them into smoothies. If you have a high-power blender, you can actually add whole nuts and they will blend without difficulty. Nuts have a high oil content, which means they can oxidize (become rancid) from heat and air exposure. Store them in airtight containers and they will stay fresh for weeks. They will also stay fresh for months when stored in food storage bags in the freezer.

APPLE

Apples contain several health-promoting nutrients that make them ideal for smoothies. They provide quercetin, which is a flavonoid that helps clear the body of environmental chemicals such as the toxin Bisphenol A (BPA). This is significant, as researchers have discovered that BPA may be a causative factor in obesity. Apples also provide malic acid, tartaric acid and lots of detoxifying soluble fiber, such as pectin. Several recent studies have found that those who eat apples daily have increased levels of healthy antioxidant enzymes, such as glutathione peroxidase, in their blood. These enzymes protect the body from environmental toxins that are linked to obesity.

Preparation and storage: Buy fresh, organic apples that are grown without chemicals. Apples have remained on the Environmental Working Group's (EWG.org) "Dirty Dozen" list for many years, as they have a higher pesticide residue than other produce. Remove the core and the stem, leaving the skin intact. Whole fresh apples last for months when stored in a cool, dark place. Just be sure they don't freeze, which damages the fruit and makes it mushy when thawed. Apples that have been cut into can be stored in a covered, airtight, glass container for up to a week in the refrigerator.

APRICOT

Rich in beta-carotene and fiber, apricots are sweet and slightly tart with a flavor that tastes like a mix of peach and plum. If you don't have apricots, use other stone fruits, such as nectarines, peaches, cherries or plums.

Preparation and storage: Remove the pit (stone), but the skin does not need to be removed. Apricots can be stored intact (with the pit) for several days without refrigeration. Once the pit is removed, they can be stored in a covered, airtight, glass container for several more days in the refrigerator. To store longer than 3 or 4 days, it's best to pit and freeze them in a wax paper bag.

AVOCADO

Avocados contain healthful fats that help reduce cholesterol levels. They provide 35% more potassium than a banana and vitamins K, B_6, B_5, C and E. They are high in calories, so use just one quarter of an avocado per serving.

Preparation and storage: Cut the avocado in half and gently twist it to separate the two halves. Leave the pit in the unused portion. Scoop out the amount of avocado to be used for your smoothie from the other half. Store the unused portion in a wax paper bag in the fridge for up to 3 days. When ready to use the other half, remove it from the storage bag and remove the pit by sticking it with a knife blade and gently twisting. If the surface of the avocado is discolored or dry, simply cut a thin slice off the top layer to reveal the fresh avocado beneath.

BANANA

Bananas are the perfect smoothie ingredient, as they blend well and provide a creamy texture, especially when frozen. They are an excellent source of potassium, B_6 (which protects against insomnia and irritability) and fructooligosaccharide (which is a prebiotic substance that encourages the growth of the healthy bacteria in the digestive system). They also contain pectin, a soluble fiber that helps promote better digestion and alleviates constipation.

Preparation and storage: Keep fresh, organic bananas on hand for smoothies. If your bananas are green or do not peel easily, they are not ripe yet. Once they have ripened to the stage where they are a uniform yellow color, they can be peeled and broken in half, and then used in your smoothie or placed in a wax paper bag to be frozen. They will keep for up to 3 months in the freezer.

BASIL

Common basil or sweet basil is different from the medicinally potent holy basil, which is an Indian culinary herb (see the "Holy Basil" entry later in this chapter). Fresh basil leaves blend well and give smoothies an herbal scent.

Preparation and storage: Dried basil leaves are available in the bulk section of many grocery stores, they last for months in an airtight glass jar and can be used if you have a high-powder blender. Fresh basil leaves are preferable as they are rich in oils that contain their healthful antioxidants, they're tender and blend well, and they add intense flavor and fragrance to smoothies. Use fresh leaves when possible. If purchased attached to their stem, they can be stored in a glass of fresh water like fresh cut flowers. If you have fresh leaves, they can be wrapped in a damp, clean tea towel and stored in the crisper drawer for about 4 days.

BEET

Cooked beets provide a rich red color and are a decent source of folate. Beets have a strong flavor that may override all other ingredients, so use them sparingly.

Preparation and storage: Washed and peeled raw beets, beet juice, and beet greens can be added to smoothies. All can be stored for up to a week in the refrigerator.

BERRIES

Berries are juicy and sweeten other smoothie ingredients when blended with them. Berries are a good source of fiber, vitamins C and E, minerals selenium and calcium, and have only around 40 calories in a ½ cup.

Blueberries provide manganese, vitamin C, vitamin K and are a rich source of anthocyanins which help reduce inflammation. They taste sweet but actually have a very low glycemic score which means they have little effect on blood sugar levels and are an excellent choice for those with diabetes. Blueberry juice works well in smoothies as does blueberry nectar, which contains more pulp, fiber and flavor than the juice and can sometimes be used in place of blueberry juice in recipes.

Raspberries contain raspberry ketone, which is a natural plant nutrient that may promote "lipolysis," the technical term for body fat breakdown and release.

Bilberries are similar to blueberries, and they are a rich source of flavonoids and vitamin C. Their deep purple pigment contains anthocyanins, which reduce inflammation and provide some protection against the aging effects of our environment.

Blackberries also contain anthocyanins and ellagic acid, which are powerful anti-cancer nutrients. They're loaded with fiber, about 8 grams per cup, and their polyphenol antioxidants help us lose weight as they fuel metabolic processes.

Preparation and storage: Use fresh berries when available and store them in the freezer. Frozen berries are ideal as they provide a rich, thick, frosty texture to smoothies. Prepackaged frozen berries, such as cherries, are also pre-pitted for ease of use in smoothies.

BLACK PEPPER

Black pepper adds some heat to smoothies. Piperine, the active ingredient in black pepper, boosts turmeric's anti-inflammatory action by up to 2000% by increasing the bioavailability of curcumin. Freshly ground black pepper is also an excellent source of potassium.

Preparation and storage: Whole peppercorns can be kept in a pepper grinder (pepper mill) and freshly ground as needed, which preserves the medicinal properties of the oils.

BLUEBERRIES

Laboratory studies have found that common blueberries (cultivated) reduce the inflammation that promotes insulin resistance, thus providing some protection against metabolic syndrome, type 2 diabetes and hypoglycemia. Blueberries add flavor, anthocyanin color, 4 grams of fiber and only 80 calories per cup.

Wild blueberries contain a higher concentration of antioxidants, and they are my favorite smoothie ingredient because they are sweet, rich in flavor and naturally contain high concentrations of health-promoting phenolic compounds. Studies have found that those who eat wild blueberries daily have lower insulin resistance as well as less weight gain and lower incidence of type 2 diabetes.

Preparation and storage: You can pick your own wild blueberries and use them fresh or freeze them. Otherwise, both wild blueberries and cultivated blueberries can be purchased in the freezer section of most grocery stores. I keep my freezer stocked with wild blueberries so that I always have some on hand for my daily smoothie.

CARAMBOLA

Yellow and waxy, carambola—also known as star fruit—is a sweet and tannic fruit that is an excellent smoothie ingredient. Carambola provides antioxidants, potassium, vitamin C and polyphenolic compounds. It is available at specialty markets and occasionally in the produce section of grocery stores.

Preparation and storage: Carambola can be added directly to smoothies, so there is no need to peel first. Carambola is a tropical fruit that should be used fresh and not frozen. No preparation is necessary as the seeds are small and the skin is soft enough to blend easily. Look for yellow starfruit, which are at the peak of ripeness but without brown spots, which indicate they may be too ripe. Starfruit that has been cut into can be stored in a covered, airtight container in the refrigerator for up to a week.

CARROT JUICE

Carrot juice is the juice of pulverized carrots. It's sweet and rich in nutrients such as beta carotene, in B vitamins such as folate, and in minerals such as calcium, magnesium, potassium and iron.

Preparation and storage: Carrot juice can be made at home with a juicer, but you'll need 1 pound of carrots to prepare 1 cup of juice, so most people opt to purchase carrot juice. Ideally, the juice should be consumed the same day, but fresh-made carrot juice lasts for just a few days in the refrigerator. Bottled carrot juice is available in most grocery stores and lasts for about a week once it's been opened.

CHERRIES

Sweet, tart, dark and sour cherries all contain anthocyanins and proanthocyanidins that help reduce inflammation and thus reduce water weight. A daily dose of cherry juice is a good idea, as evidence is accumulating that glucaric acid, found in cherries, has a role in the prevention and nutritional treatment of cancer. Cherries also provide melatonin and tryptophan, which support proper sleep and those who get proper sleep lose more body fat and keep it off.

Preparation and storage: Fresh cherries must be pitted; therefore, it's easier to buy pre-pitted frozen cherries. Cherry juice and black cherry concentrate are available in the juice section of the grocery store.

CHIA SEEDS

These little seeds are similar to hemp seeds and flaxseeds. They're tiny nutrition packets of protein, fiber and omega-3 fatty acids. They provide 6 grams of fiber, 3 grams of omega-3 fatty acids and 3 grams of protein in just 1 tablespoon.

Preparation and storage: Chia seeds are available at Trader Joe's, food co-ops, grocery stores that sell Bob's Red Mill products and online. They come in resealable plastic food storage bags and can be stored in an airtight glass container in a cupboard or in the freezer. Chia seeds blend well in smoothies, but they can also be ground into a powder in a coffee grinder. Chia powder blends completely into smoothies, which may be preferable to the whole seeds for those sensitive to certain textures. Seeds generally have a high oil content and will keep longer in the freezer.

CHILI PEPPERS

Chili peppers contain capsaicinoids and carotenoids, groups of natural compounds that promote weight loss. These hot peppers add zest to cold drinks. They add a depth to the flavor and a little heat on the back of the tongue. Try a small amount the first time you're making a hot pepper smoothie and adjust according to your taste.

Preparation and storage: Remove the stem and the seeds, and taste your pepper to make sure it's not too hot before adding it to your smoothie. Fresh hot peppers can be stored for up to a week in the refrigerator.

CHOCOLATE
(See the entry for "Cocoa Powder.")

CILANTRO
Cilantro leaves provide fresh flavor and fragrance to smoothies. The seeds of the cilantro plant, commonly known as coriander, have a lemony citrus flavor due to the linalool, a natural terpene that is a precursor to vitamin E.

Preparation and storage: Rinse cilantro leaves and chop lightly before adding to smoothies. If you are using a high-power blender, you can use the cilantro stems as well. The best way to store cilantro is to rinse it well and while still wet wrap it in a clean tea towel and store in the crisper drawer of your refrigerator for up to a week. If your cilantro is starting to look droopy or dried out, simply cut off the bottoms of the stems and place them in a glass of fresh water just as you would to bring back a bouquet of flowers. The stalks of cilantro should perk up within a few hours at which time the whole bunch can be rinsed in fresh water and stored as above.

CINNAMON
True cinnamon is from the inner bark of Cinnamomum trees, but a majority of the cinnamon we buy is actually from the cassia tree. It contains strong oils, so a little goes a long way in terms of flavor. Recent studies have demonstrated

that cinnamon polyphenols help repair pancreatic beta cells in diabetic mice.

Preparation and storage: Ground cinnamon is widely available. If your cinnamon powder has been in your cupboard for a while and has lost its flavor, it has also lost its nutritional effectiveness. Just toss it and buy some new ground cinnamon. Store cinnamon powder in a glass airtight container and out of the light if possible.

CITRUS

Citrus fruits provide vitamin C and bioflavonoids as well as fiber. The younger and fresher the fruit, the more easily it will blend. Citrus fruits such as kumquats, blood oranges, Mandarin oranges, navel oranges, clementines, lemons, limes, grapefruits and tangerines are delicious additions to smoothies.

Blood oranges are colorful and sweet, and they are a rich source of the antioxidant pigment anthocyanin, vitamin C, calcium, folate and thiamine. Clementines are a variety of the Mandarin orange and are ideal for smoothies because they're easy to peel, seedless and sweet. Meyer lemons, a cross between an orange and a lemon, smell heavenly, and their juice is a little sweeter and less tart than other lemons.

Preparation and storage: Citrus fruits must be peeled before adding them to a blender. The bioflavonoids can be retained by using a knife to cut away the colorful and tough outer part of the skin, leaving the pithy white part intact. Toss the segments with the pith intact into smoothies. Fresh oranges keep for up to a week in the refrigerator and up to three weeks in the freezer. Once peeled or cut into, they should be stored in a wax paper bag and can be kept refrigerated for up to 4 days.

COCOA POWDER

Cocoa contains a nutrient called epicatechin that induces lipolysis, which helps our bodies release stored fat, especially around the stomach and abdomen. Its flavonols have been found to prevent diabetes in animal studies (though not in human studies yet), and it helps reduce our need for insulin.

Preparation and storage: Look for unsweetened organic cocoa powder. It will last for months in a covered container.

COCONUT

Fresh coconut—including the meat, milk and water—is ideal for smoothie making. I don't have access to fresh coconut except when I'm traveling, so I buy dried organic coconut flakes and ground macaroon coconut online from Bob's Red Mill.

Ground coconut adds tropical flavor, a little texture, and considerable minerals and fiber to smoothies. Coconut milk adds a richness to smoothies, and the cultured coconut milk products provide health-supportive probiotics. Coconut water has a sweet, nutty flavor and provides trace minerals (electrolytes) such as sodium, magnesium and manganese, as well as concentrated amounts of potassium. It's naturally low in fat, calories and sugar, so it's an ideal weight-loss smoothie base liquid.

Preparation and storage: I don't recommend preparing fresh coconut unless you have exeprience with it, as it's fairly involved. However, coconut milk, cultured coconut milk and coconut water are all available in most grocery stores and online. They last for about a week in the refrigerator once opened.

COCONUT PALM NECTAR

Coconut palm nectar is a sweetener made from the sap of cut flower buds from the coconut palm. When we think of coconut products we generally think of the coconut's water, milk or meat, but this product is different as it is made from the coconut palm flowers. It is specifically used as a sweetener and is showing promise as a sweetener for those needing to balance blood sugar and those who want to lose weight because it does not appear to spike blood sugar levels the way most carb-based sweeteners do. It is nutrient dense, high in potassium and magnesium, and is low glycemic. It provides a mellow, sweet flavor and dissolves well in smoothies.

Preparation and storage: Coconut palm nectar is available in a syrup form, which must be refrigerated once opened, or dry as granules, which is stored like other granulated sugars in an air- and moisture-tight container.

COFFEE

Coffee is the number one source of antioxidants for Americans because it's such a popular drink and so much is consumed. And any food or drink we consume daily is going to have an impact on our health, so it's important to buy organic coffee in order to reduce exposure to pesticides. Coffee contains polyphenol compounds that are being studied for their ability to improve metabolic syndrome, a condition that affects an estimated 25% of the US population. Researchers believe that the polyphenol antioxidants improve the way our bodies use insulin. Keep in mind that probiotics in the digestive tract are neccesary for the absorption of these polyphenols. So eating yogurt or taking a probiotic supplement is a good idea. Coffee extracts, such as manno-oligosaccharides, are also being studied for their potential as weight-loss nutrients.

Preparation and storage: Use organic, freshly brewed coffee or instant coffee in smoothies. Instant coffee is simply freeze-dried coffee; it has a long shelf life and can be stored in the freezer for up to a year. Freeze-dried coffee crystals are ideal as they dissolve well in smoothies. Decaffeinated instant coffee is also available for those who want the coffee flavor without the caffeine. If you're making freshly brewed coffee from whole coffee beans, the beans can be stored in the freezer, whether they're whole or ground, and they will stay fresh for months. Brewed coffee can be kept in a glass container in the refrigerator for up to a week.

COTTAGE CHEESE

Cottage cheese is a high-protein food, containing 14 grams per each ½ cup. It also contains nutrients that stimulate the release of a hunger-fighting hormone called peptide YY, reducing appetite and helping weight loss. It becomes cream-like in a blender and mixes well with other smoothie ingredients.

Preparation and storage: Buy only organic cottage cheese to avoid hormones and chemicals. Once opened, it keeps for up to a week in the refrigerator.

CRANBERRIES

Cranberries are tart and almost bitter and beg for a little sweetener, which can add calories to a smoothie. Therefore, whole cranberries and cranberry juice should be used sparingly and combined with sweeter fruits to mellow their intensity. Cranberries contain proanthocyanidins that keep bacteria from sticking to the urinary tract, thus their benefit in reducing urinary tract infections.

Preparation and storage: Fresh cranberries are only available in the winter, and can be stored in an airtight container in the refrigerator for up to 2 months. However, canned and frozen cranberries are available year round. Cranberry concentrate and cranberry juice are both widely available.

CUCUMBER

Cucumbers are low calorie and provide electrolytes, and their flavor blends well with fruits and vegetables, making them an ideal smoothie ingredient.

Preparation and storage: Peel the skin off cucumbers before adding to smoothies. Since cucumbers are highly sprayed with pesticides, buy organic cucumbers as they are grown without chemicals. Buy fresh cucumbers that are firm and without blemishes or soft spots. Store them in the crisper drawer of the refrigerator. Once cut into, cucumber can be stored in a covered, airtight, glass container for about 4 days.

EXTRACTS AND OILS

Flavor extracts can add a lot of flavor and scent to a smoothie with just a few drops. For example, orange oil or vanilla, hazelnut and almond extracts provide flavor without the calories and carbs.

Preparation and storage: Extracts are available at most grocery stores and have a long shelf life.

FIBER

Foods high in fiber as well as fiber supplements, such as acacia fiber (gum arabic) and glucomannan (konjac root), help us feel full and reduce our appetite. Studies have found that fiber supports weight loss and lowers blood cholesterol.

Preparation and storage: Fiber powders are available from supplement manufacturers, at food co-ops and supplement stores. They are sold in individual packets or in airtight containers and when kept dry and cool, will stay fresh for months. Be consistent with the amount you use daily so that your body can adjust to your water needs when taking fiber supplements.

FIG

Figs act as a sweetener for smoothies and are a great source of fiber, potassium, manganese and vitamin B_6.

Preparation and storage: With fresh figs, remove the stem and rinse under water, and then drop them into smoothies whole. Fresh figs can be kept in an airtight container in the refrigerator but they only last for about 2 days. They can also be sliced and frozen. Dried figs have a longer shelf life (1 month), especially when refrigerated (6 months). Both fresh and dried figs work well in smoothies. If you're using a high-power blender, dried figs will blend easily. However, some blenders are not able to completely break down dried fruits. If your blender is lower powered, you might opt for fresh figs, which blend much more easily.

FISH OIL

A Brazilian lab study found that fish oil improves glucose tolerance and weight loss. Orange-flavored fish oil tastes delicious and can be added to smoothies to boost dietary essential fatty acids.

Preparation and storage: Keep all fish oils refrigerated. Add up to 1 teaspoon to your smoothies per day.

FLAXSEED MEAL

Flaxseed meal is simply ground flaxseed. Since the seeds are difficult to chew, ground flaxseed is a better option for smoothies. Flaxseeds contain essential fatty acids, but note that they also contain phytoestrogens, which can cause a hormonal imbalance for some. Other essential fatty acid sources that do not affect hormones are avocado, hemp seeds, chia seeds and borage oil.

Preparation and storage: Whole flaxseeds and flaxseed meal are available in most grocery stores. Their oils are delicate and oxidize easily from heat and oxygen. Store them in an airtight container in the freezer, and they will last for months.

GARLIC

Garlic supports the endocrine system and improves thyroid function, thus increasing metabolism. Garlic also contains over 400 different compounds that kill bacteria, viruses and fungi.

Preparation and storage: Peel the skin from a clove of garlic and chop it so it doesn't get caught under the blender blades. Peeled garlic cloves can be stored in an airtight container in the refrigerator for several weeks.

GINGER

Ginger root is full of flavor, fiber and active compounds that reduce inflammation and nausea. Pickled ginger, powdered dried ginger (available in the spice section of the grocery store) or ginger juice can all be used in place of fresh ginger root. However, fresh ginger tastes better, provides more fiber and contains nutrients that support weight loss.

Preparation and storage: Fresh ginger root is available in the produce department of most grocery stores. Use a knife to remove the outside skin and then chop off about 1 inch of root (about a tablespoon). If you have a high-power blender, you may be able to use the ginger without peeling. Fresh ginger root lasts for about a week in a cool, dry place such as the crisper drawer of your refrigerator. To keep ginger fresh longer, store the unpeeled root in a wax paper bag in the freezer where it will stay fresh for months. When you need fresh ginger, you can pull it out of the freezer, grate some into your recipe and then return the root to the freezer. The peel will grate easily when frozen.

GRAPES

Grapes are very sweet, so a small amount adds a lot of flavor. They also add powerful anti-inflammatory nutrients, such as anthocyanins and resveratrol, to smoothies.

Preparation and storage: Freeze whole seedless grapes so you'll have some of these delicious little flavor packs on hand when you need to sweeten up a smoothie. It is also possible to use grapes that have seeds, but seedless grapes make for a smoother, preferable smoothie texture.

GREEK YOGURT

For centuries, the Greeks have strained their yogurt to remove extra liquid, which increases the amount of protein by weight. Greek yogurt has roughly twice as much protein as ordinary yogurt and it's delicious!

Preparation and storage: Read yogurt labels and look for organic products with no added sugar or food coloring. Look for nonfat yogurt to replicate the recipes in this book. Taste-test yogurts until you find the brand you like best, and then stick with it. I like Green Valley Organics yogurt, as it's lactose-free, as well as FAGE Total 0% nonfat Greek yogurt, as they have a creamy texture, are low in sugar, contain no chemicals and are high in protein. Yogurt can be kept in the fridge for about 5 days once it's been opened.

GREEN TEA

Green tea has become a popular health food for its epigallocatechin gallate (EGCG) polyphenol, as this supports the production of the weight-loss hormone noradrenaline. This hormone increases fat burning and modulates dietary fat absorption and metabolism.

Preparation and storage: The trick with green tea is to steep it lightly, which will infuse your water with all the polyphenol nutrients before the bitter substances have a chance to be absorbed from the leaves. To do this, simply steep tea leaves (1 tablespoon of loose leaf or 2 tea bags) for only 2 minutes in water that has just boiled but is slightly cooler than boiling temperature. Steep in a large glass pitcher. Remove tea leaves after 2 minutes, and then chill the tea in the refrigerator for up to 5 days to use in smoothies. Freeze some of your brew in ice cube trays so you'll have access to green tea even when you're too busy to brew a pot.

GREENS

Greens such as beet greens, baby spinach, baby chard, turnip greens and salad greens add fiber, minerals and fresh flavor to smoothies and pair well with fruit juice.

Preparation and storage: Buy organic greens when possible. Rinse them and wrap them in a damp, clean tea towel and store in the crisper drawer of your refrigerator for up to 3 days.

HAZELNUTS

Hazelnuts, which are also known as filberts, are flavorful and rich in calcium, unsaturated fats and B vitamins, such as thiamine and B_6. Whole nuts can be added to smoothies made in high-power blenders, or hazelnut milk can be used in smoothies to add flavor and nutrients.

Preparation and storage: You can use store-bought hazelnut milk or make your own. Freshly made hazelnut milk is incredibly delicious, and it's easy to make. Soak hazelnuts overnight in water, then pour off the soaking water and place them in a blender. Add 3 parts water to 1 part hazelnuts and blend well. Strain mixture through cheesecloth to remove the hazelnut pulp, and you have freshly made hazelnut milk. See daniellachace.com for more detailed instructions. It lasts for about 2 days when refrigerated.

HEMP SEEDS

Hemp seeds (aka hulled hemp seeds) have a mild, nut-like flavor and have a creamy texture when blended in smoothies. They're a perfect addition to smoothies because of their protein and essential fatty acids. They're rich in polyunsaturated fats that our bodies need, and we use these healthful fats in our skin, hair and body processes rather than storing them away as body fat. They're a rich source of omega-3 fatty acids and amino acids, which can improve our health when eaten daily. Two tablespoons provide 5 grams of protein.

Preparation and storage: Hulled hemp seeds and hemp seed protein are available from Bob's Red Mill in most grocery stores as well as online. They're ready to eat right out of the package. No prep necessary. Just pour them into your smoothie. They can be stored in the freezer for up to a year.

HERBAL TEA

Herbal tea makes a wonderful base for smoothies. Brew a batch of your favorite herbal tea, such as peppermint or chamomile. My favorite herbal blend is called Bengal Spice and it was created by Charlie Baden, the culinary blendmaster at Celestial Seasonings. It's a caffeine free, chai-type, blend and it makes a wonderful smoothie base.

Preparation and storage: Pour brewed tea into ice cube trays and freeze. Once frozen, keep the ice cubes in a sealed bag in the freezer and use them as desired for smoothies to add flavor and fragrance without calories, sugar or fat.

HOLY BASIL

Holy basil, also known as Tulsi in Ayurvedic medicine, contains oleanolic acid, a powerful immune-supportive nutrient. In studies of mice, the ursolic acid in holy basil has been shown to increase muscle and reduce fat (obesity). It also contains rosmarinic acid, a natural phenolic that supports metabolism and reduces inflammation.

Preparation and storage: Holy basil plants can be grown in your garden or in pots on a porch. Fresh holy basil is available in some grocery stores in the produce section, and dried holy basil is available in the bulk section of many grocery stores. If your local market does not yet carry holy basil, you may want to request it, as it is available through bulk suppliers such as Frontier. To keep basil stalks fresh, trim the stems and place them in a glass of fresh water and keep them out on the counter just as you would fresh flowers.

ICE

Ice cubes give smoothies a frosty texture. Filtering tap water that is used for ice will remove chlorine, and if you have a solid carbon filter, it will also remove heavy metals and other chemicals. This improves the flavor of the ice cubes and protects you from environmental toxins.

Preparation and storage: Filter tap water before pouring into ice cube trays or hook up a filtration system to your automatic ice maker. Store-bought ice is usually not filtered.

KIWI

Kiwi fruit provide vitamin C and a tart flavor but are often sour unless you are able to get them locally and ripe off the vine. Balance the sour flavor with sweet fruit, such as berries.

Preparation and storage: Fresh, ripe kiwi can be used with skin intact in high-power blenders. However, some blenders have a hard time with kiwi skin, in which case the skin can be removed by cutting a kiwi in half and using a spoon to scoop out the green flesh. Store unused kiwi in an airtight container in the refrigerator for up to a week.

MANGO

Fresh mango is rich in skin-protecting carotenoids and fiber. The flesh is sweet and has an exotic flavor. When frozen, mango adds a creamy, frosty texture to smoothies.

Preparation and storage: The skin and pit must be removed from fresh mangoes before adding to the blender. Frozen mango is ideal, as it has been pre-chopped and the pit and skin have been removed. Unripe mangoes can be kept at room temperature for up to a week as they ripen. Once ripe, they can be stored in the refrigerator for up to 2 weeks. When they've reached their peak ripeness, remove the skin and the pit and chop the sweet yellow fruit, which can then be stored in a wax paper bag and frozen for months.

MELONS

Honeydew, cantaloupe, watermelon, crenshaw and other melons are all delicious additions to smoothies. They provide provitamin-A substances, electrolytes and antioxidants to smoothies with a lot of sweet flavor.

Preparation and storage: Remove the rind and seeds and use fresh, or chop and freeze for later use.

MILK

Dairy milk provides protein and gives smoothies a milkshake texture. Goat's milk can also be used, and for those who are vegan or lactose intolerant, there are many additional dairy milk alternatives, such as hazelnut, almond (see the "Almond Milk" entry), rice, hemp or coconut milk.

Preparation and storage: Buy organic milk when possible to avoid hormones such as bovine growth hormone, and to avoid pesticide and herbicide residue. Milk is usually good for about a week after the sell-by expiration date that is stamped on the product.

MINT

Fresh mint leaves contain oils that provide intense flavor. Use sparingly, as they dramatically change the flavor of smoothies.

Preparation and storage: Fresh mint leaves are sold in the produce department of the grocery store. Rinse and add directly to smoothies. Keep mint stalks fresh by cutting off the bottom inch of the stems, which allows them to take up fresh water. Then place them in a glass of fresh water just as you would with cut flowers where they will stay fresh at room temperature for up to a week. Be sure to keep the water fresh by changing it daily. If you've already removed the leaves from the stalks, the leaves can be rinsed and rolled up in a clean tea towel and stored in the crisper drawer of the refrigerator for about a week.

NECTARINE

(See the entry for "Stone Fruit.")

NUTMEG

Nutmeg contains essential oils that provide flavor and fragrance and may improve digestion.

Preparation and storage: Buy whole nutmeg and grate fresh as needed to preserve the oils. Ground nutmeg is available in the spice section of the grocery store and in bulk. It is rich in oils that oxidize from light, air and heat so keep it in an airtight container and in a cool, dark place. Ground nutmeg will retain its flavor and fragrance for up to a year when stored properly.

PEANUT BUTTER

Peanut butter is a rich source of the amino acid leucine, which plays a role in preserving muscle mass during weight loss and also increases the rate of metabolism and fat burning.

Preparation and storage: Some of the high-power blenders have the ability to turn whole peanuts into peanut butter. Fresh ground peanut butter can be purchased at many co-ops and whole food stores. If you are buying pre-made peanut butter, look for products made with only peanuts—no sugar, no hydrogenated oils and no preservatives. Be on the lookout for peanut butter varieties labeled "aflatoxin-free," as they are the least allergenic. Peanut butter can be stored for about a month at room temperature but should be kept in a cool, dark place such as a pantry or cupboard. Peanut butter will stay fresh for about a year in the refrigerator.

PEAR

Most pears taste great in smoothies. Asian pears are especially sweet and juicy and provide ample fiber.

Preparation and storage: Remove core and blend. Pears ripen quickly and only last for a few days once they're cut into. Store unused, cut pears in the refrigerator for up to 3 days.

PINEAPPLE

Fresh pineapple is intensely sweet when ripe and adds a heady, tropical aroma to smoothies. Pineapple juice contains bromelain, which reduces inflammation and aids in digestion.

Preparation and storage: Remove the skin and core of fresh pineapple, or use canned pineapple or pineapple juice. Store pineapple in a glass container with a lid for up to 3 days in the refrigerator. I use frozen pineapple that is sold in the freezer section of most grocery stores specifically for smoothies. It's sweet and ripe and flash-frozen so the individual pieces pour out easily into the blender.

POMEGRANATE

Pomegranate seeds (arils) are jewel-like in appearance and juicy. They are nutritious and provide vitamin C, vitamin K and free-radical scavenging polyphenols (ellagitannins and flavonoids).

Preparation and storage: Whole seeds can be purchased in the freezer section of most grocery stores and are much easier to use than a whole pomegranate, which you'll need to mine for its seeds. If you opt for using a fresh whole pomegranate, the whole fruit will last for 2–3 weeks at room temperature and up to 2 months in the refrigerator. You'll need to cut the fruit into quarters and carefully pull the seeds out of the white material. Collect the seeds in a bowl and when you have about ¼ cup, pour them into your smoothie. Pomegranate juice and pomegranate concentrate are also available in the juice section of the grocery store.

PROBIOTICS

Probiotics are supplements that contain healthy bacteria that adhere to our intestinal lining, where they help us with digestion and detoxification and support the metabolism of phytochemicals in our digestive tract. Probiotics support weight loss. Researchers are discovering that there is a correlation between higher levels of gut flora (probiotics and prebiotics) in our digestive tracts and weight loss.

Preparation and storage: Most probiotic supplements must be stored in the refrigerator. Buy powdered probiotic supplements, as they are easier to add to smoothies. Many probiotic supplements sold in capsules can be opened and their powdery contents poured into your smoothie. (See my website at daniellachace.com for recommendations.)

PROTEIN POWDERS

Pea, rice, soy, hemp and whey protein powders add concentrated protein to smoothies. A Purdue University study found that diets higher in protein may help preserve lean body mass, which is the best fat burner of all. Studies also show that increasing protein reduces the appetite and sugar cravings.

Preparation and storage: Spiru-Tein Vanilla is one of my favorite protein powders, as it has a creamy texture and it's low in sugar. MediClear Plus by Thorne Research is a rice-based protein powder that provides 32 grams of protein per serving, and it contains nutrients that help reduce inflammation. Protein powders are available in grocery stores, health food stores and online. (See my website at daniel-lachace.com for other recommendations.) Protein powders can be stored at room temperature for several weeks but they stay fresh for months when stored in the freezer. They can be stored in their original containers as long as they have an airtight lid.

PRUNE

Dried plums are called prunes. They're sweet and full of fiber, so they're an excellent sweetener for weight-loss smoothies.

Preparation and storage: Pre-pitted prunes are the easiest to use for smoothies, and they last for several months in an airtight container.

PUMPKIN

Fresh cooked pumpkin adds cancer-fighting mixed carotenoids and fiber to smoothies.

Preparation and storage: If you happen to have fresh cooked pumpkin on hand, certainly try it in a smoothie; otherwise, just buy canned pumpkin, which is already cooked and ready to use. Cooked pumpkin or leftover canned pumpkin can be stored in a covered, airtight, glass container in the refrigerator for up to a week and in the freezer for months.

PUMPKIN SEEDS

Pumpkin seeds are one of our richest vegan food sources of the mineral zinc. Zinc reduces cravings and improves insulin's effectiveness.

Preparation and storage: Pumpkin seeds are sold in the bulk department and in the baking aisle of most grocery stores. Add a tablespoon to smoothies if you have a high-power blender that can break down the fiber in these seeds. If your blender is not able to grind seeds well, they can be ground in a coffee grinder and stored in a glass container in the freezer for up to 6 months.

PURIFIED WATER

(See the entry for "Ice.") Purified tap water can be used in smoothies and to make ice cubes. Purifying with a solid carbon filter at the tap removes toxins such as heavy metals as well as chlorine. Therefore, filtering water detoxifies it as well as improves its flavor and smell.

SESAME SEEDS

Sesame seeds are an excellent source of the amino acid leucine, which plays a role in preserving muscle mass during weight loss and raising the metabolism and fat-burning rate.

Preparation and storage: Whole, shelled sesame seeds or sesame seed butter, also known as tahini, can be added to smoothies to boost protein. Add only 1 tablespoon, as sesame seeds contain natural oils that are dense in calories. Tahini lasts for about a year in the refrigerator.

SPARKLING WATER

I drink sparkling mineral water such as San Pellegrino because I feel hydrated from the water's minerals and I find the bubbles refreshing. I love to add it to fruit (non-cream based) smoothies after they've been blended, and have recommended adding sparkling water to smoothie recipes throughout the recipe section of this book. Add the sparkling water to the smoothie after blending all the other ingredients, as the bubbles go flat from too much blending.

Preparation and storage: I buy a couple of cases of San Pellegrino when I'm at Costco and keep it in the pantry so that I always have some on hand. It lasts for about a year when unopened. Once opened the bubbles begin to dissipate and the carbonation is lost within a day, so it's best to drink it within a few hours.

STAR FRUIT

(See the entry for "Carambola.")

STONE FRUIT

Nectarines, peaches, donut peaches, apricots and plums are all stone fruit, and they're all excellent smoothie ingredients. They provide the usual fiber, vitamins and a whole lot of sweet flavor.

Preparation and storage: Always buy organic peaches and nectarines, as non-organic varieties are typically highly sprayed with chemical pesticides. The skin can be left on when adding to smoothies, but the pit must be removed from stone fruits. They can be pitted and then frozen or you can find pre-pitted, frozen fruit for smoothie making in most grocery stores.

STRAWBERRIES

Strawberries are low on the Glycemic Index, as they contain fiber that releases their sugars slowly, thus making them a good choice for those who are balancing blood sugar, hypoglycemia or diabetes and those who want to lose weight.

Preparation and storage: Buy organic strawberries, as the conventionally grown strawberries are one of the most highly sprayed crops in the United States. Fresh strawberries need their green top leaves removed, but leave the seeds and skin intact when adding to smoothies. Frozen strawberries provide a frosty texture to smoothies and they're easy to keep on hand, as they last for about a year in the freezer.

SWEETENERS

Sweeteners are rarely needed in smoothies and some can add calories, so it's a good idea to keep them to a minimum. Whole fruits and dried fruits such as dates can be used to add sweetness instead—they naturally contain fiber, which gives them a lower glycemic load.

Honey and agave nectar are liquid sugars. These syrups are flavorful, so a little goes a long way. The addition of these insulin-stimulating sugars should be minimized. Try to use them only when needed (for example, in a particularly bitter recipe, such as one with grapefruit juice or pomegranate seeds).

Also, go easy on the sweeteners that don't have fiber such as sugar (this also applies to honey and agave nectar). A better alternative is coconut palm nectar, as it is a low-glycemic sweetener that comes in the form of syrup or crystals. Its Glycemic Index is only 35 compared to honey at 55 to 83, and sugar at 65 to 100. Coconut palm nectar also has less than 20% fructose compared to agave at 55% to 95% and high-fructose corn syrup at 55%. Still, use only about a teaspoon of coconut palm nectar in a smoothie.

Avoid synthetic chemical sweeteners such as Equal (aspartame), saccharin, Splenda (sucralose) and NutraSweet (aspartame), as studies have proven that they increase weight gain, cause headaches and contribute to joint pain, and many of them increase the risk for cancer.

Alcohol sugars, such as xylitol, erythritol and maltitol, are very sweet and nontoxic. They don't raise blood sugar levels because they're not easily absorbed into the bloodstream, so they don't stimulate insulin production. Just a teaspoon of xylitol will take the edge off a blender full of bitter or sour produce. Alcohol sweeteners also provide some health benefits, such as reducing dental cavities and feeding flora in the digestive system. Coconut palm nectar is showing promise in new studies as a low-glycemic alternative sweetener.

Preparation and storage: Liquid sweeteners can be stored in the cupboard for months and refrigeration extends their shelf life even further. Coconut palm nectar is sold as granulated sugar and as a syrup. Xylitol and erythritol are sold as granules, and maltitol is available as a powder or syrup.

TURMERIC

Turmeric is a root grown in south Asia that is ground and used extensively as a culinary and medicinal spice. It has a mild, bitter flavor and is an ideal addition to all weight-loss smoothies, as it helps reduce the water weight that causes cellulite. Turmeric contains an active compound called curcumin, a powerful anti-inflammatory agent. Turmeric is used in India as part of the daily diet to prevent edema and inflammation.

Preparation and storage: Buy ground turmeric powder and store it in an airtight container. Be careful when handling turmeric powder, as the yellow color stains cloth and some countertop materials.

UNSWEETENED COCOA POWDER

(See the entry for "Cocoa Powder.")

WHEY

Whey is a good source of protein and makes us feel full. Studies have found that whey protein powder promotes a reduction in adipose tissue (body fat). Other studies have determined that consuming 1 to 2 grams of whey protein per 2.2 pounds of body weight per day, in conjunction with strength training, may improve lean body mass.

Preparation and storage: Protein powders can be stored in the freezer to extend their shelf life for up to a year. Jarrow Organic Whey Protein Powder and Nature's Plus Spiru-Tein have a creamy texture that is great for smoothies.

XYLITOL

Xylitol is a low-calorie alcohol sweetener. A recent South African study from the University of Kwa Zulu-Natal found that xylitol can be used not only as a sugar substitute but also as a supplement for those with diabetes. It has a cool flavor and dissolves well.

Preparation and storage: Xylitol granules can be stored in a cupboard for about a year.

CHAPTER 3

The Smoothie Maker's Kitchen

This chapter provides the shopping lists for smoothie ingredients, tips for prepping them and a review of the basic kitchen tools needed for smoothie making. When shopping for smoothie ingredients, choose a few items from each category to stock your pantry. That way you'll be able to make smoothies in minutes, right when you're craving them, without having to make a trip to the store. Most of the ingredients listed below can be stored in a pantry or freezer for months.

MILKS AND WATERS

Coconut water is an excellent smoothie liquid, as it's low in calories and rich in electrolytes. Milk alternatives and coconut water are available in aspetic boxes that can be stored, unopened and unrefrigerated, for months.

» Almond milk

» Coconut milk

» Coconut water

» Cultured coconut milk

» Hazelnut milk

» Hemp milk

» Kefir

» Oat milk

» Rice milk

» Sparkling water

NECTARS AND JUICES

Fruit juices in glass bottles can be stored, unopened and unrefrigerated, for up to a year. Grab a few bottles of your favorite juices when they're on sale and store them in a cupboard so you'll have them on hand. Nectars have a richer flavor and more pulp than juices, however, and therefore are ideal for smoothies.

- » Apricot nectar
- » Black cherry concentrate
- » Black currant nectar
- » Blueberry nectar
- » Carrot juice
- » Cherry juice
- » Cranberry concentrate
- » Grapefruit juice
- » Lemon juice
- » Lime juice
- » Mango nectar
- » Orange juice
- » Papaya nectar
- » Peach nectar
- » Pineapple juice
- » Pomegranate concentrate
- » Pomegranate juice
- » Prune juice
- » Tangerine juice
- » Tomato juice
- » Unfiltered apple juice

FROZEN FRUITS

Frozen berries and fruits are sold in bags in the freezer section of most stores explicitly for smoothie making. They're wonderful because the berries are pre-pitted; fruits such as mangoes, peaches and pineapples are chopped into small pieces that are easy on our blenders and they're generally frozen at the peak of ripeness, so the fruit is sweet and juicy.

- » Blackberries
- » Blueberries
- » Cherries
- » Cranberries
- » Dark cherries
- » Mangoes
- » Nectarines
- » Peaches
- » Pineapples
- » Raspberries
- » Strawberries
- » Sweet cherries
- » Wild blackberries
- » Wild blueberries
- » Wild huckleberries
- » Wild lingonberries

PROTEIN SUPPLEMENTS

Powders and seeds can be stored in the freezer, which helps preserve their oils and keeps them fresh longer.

- » Chia seed
- » Hemp protein powder
- » Hulled hemp seed
- » MediClear Plus protein powder
- » Organic whey powder
- » Spiru-Tein protein powder

FLAVORINGS AND SWEETENERS

Most flavorings, sweeteners and cocoa can be stored in a cool, dry place for many months, even after they've been opened. We use such small amounts of each of these products that they last a long time and are worth the investment.

- » Coconut palm nectar crystals
- » Coconut palm nectar syrup
- » Unsweetened cocoa powder
- » Vanilla beans
- » Vanilla extract
- » Xylitol

TEAS

Loose-leaf tea or tea bags can be used to brew tea for smoothies. Brew tea ahead of time and freeze it in ice cube trays, then pop the frozen tea cubes into a wax paper bag or plastic food storage bag and store for months in the freezer.

- » Bengal spice tea
- » Black tea
- » Chamomile tea
- » Green tea
- » Peppermint tea
- » White tea

COFFEES

Buy a small glass container of organic instant coffee and keep it in your freezer. It will last for a year and very little is needed—just one teaspoon per smoothie. You'll have plenty on hand for those quick morning cafe smoothies.

- » Brewed organic coffee
- » Instant coffee
- » Instant decaf coffee

FRESH FROM THE STORE AS NEEDED

The rest of the ingredients you'll need for smoothies—such as greens, fruits, veggies and yogurt—are perishables and will need to be purchased within days of use. Pick up the fresh items you'll need at your local farmers' market or in the produce section when you're at the store.

HOW TO PREP YOUR PRODUCE FOR SMOOTHIES

After shopping, spend a little time prepping produce, brewing tea ahead of time, etc., which will reduce the amount of time it takes to whip up your favorite smoothie at a moment's notice.

Peel These: Anything with a tough skin should be peeled before freezing and before adding to the blender.

- » Bananas
- » Clementines
- » Cucumbers
- » Garlic
- » Ginger root
- » Grapefruits
- » Lemons
- » Limes
- » Mandarin oranges
- » Mangoes
- » Meyer lemons
- » Oranges
- » Pineapples

Scoop These: Remove any pits or seeds; then scoop the flesh into your smoothie.

- » Avocado
- » Cantaloupe
- » Coconut
- » Honeydew melon
- » Pomegranate (use seeds only)
- » Watermelon

Pit These: Remove the pits but leave the skin intact, as most blenders can handle the delicate skin on this type of produce.

» Apricots	» Donut peaches	» Peaches
» Cherries	» Mangoes	» Plums
» Dates	» Nectarines	» Prunes

Core These: Remove the core but leave the skin intact, as most blenders can handle the skin on this type of produce.

» Apples	» Pears

Wash These: Wash greens by rinsing them under running water.

» Cilantro	» Kale	» Spinach
» Holy basil	» Mint	» Sweet basil

Freeze These: Freeze fresh berries and bananas as well as seeds so they'll last longer and provide a frosty texture to smoothies.

» Bananas	» Cherries	» Hulled Hemp Seed
» Berries	» Chia seed	

Freshly made smoothies can't be kept for long, as the ingredients break down quickly (the enzymes from the produce are released when broken down by the blender blade) and separate. But you can pour your leftover smoothie into an ice cube tray and freeze. Your smoothie cubes can be tossed back into a blender later with liquid to make a quick, thick, frosty drink with those leftovers. You can also drop them into a glass of juice or water to add flavor and electrolytes.

Grind These: Seeds and dried herbs can be pre-ground before adding to smoothies. Chia seed and flaxseed can be ground to aid in their digestion. Grinding breaks apart the hard outer casing of each little seed, which releases its healthy oils for easier absorption. In addition, if your blender is older, if the blender's blades are dull or if your blender is of a very low power, then some dried herbs may not break down well; therefore, pre-grinding them will powder those little twigs and dried leaves so they blend well when used in a smoothie.

- » Cardamom pods
- » Chia seed
- » Cinnamon sticks
- » Dried holy basil
- » Flaxseed
- » Vanilla bean
- » Whole cloves

KITCHEN TOOLS FOR SMOOTHIES

Just a few simple tools are needed to make smoothies. You'll need a blender with a strong motor and sharp blades; otherwise, your ice and tough ingredients will just bounce around in the blender's pitcher. I've tried several blenders that I feel fit the criteria:

- The **BlendTec** has a strong motor and as it is small, it fits well on my countertop. It also has clear measurement lines on the side of the pitcher, so I don't have to use a measuring cup.

- The **Tribest** is a small, single-serving blender that does a powerful job on the tough ingredients, uses a glass mason jar as the pitcher and is very inexpensive.

- The **VitaMix** has a high-power motor that easily grinds through ice, frozen fruit, nuts and other ingredients.

Opt for glass rather than plastic whenever possible to avoid the obesogenic chemicals such as BPA that can be leached from plastics into our food. Buy products in glass rather than plastic, especially those that are acidic such as juices. Choose blenders with glass pitchers, glass kitchen storage containers, glass measuring cups, etc.

I use glass containers from Crate & Barrel to store my liquids, and for the dry storage of foods, such as nuts, oatmeal and coffee, I use OXO Good Grip POP containers, which are BPA-free.

You'll also want a cutting board for prepping fruits and veggies. I'm thrilled with the Epicurean boards. I have one for meats and one for produce. I run them through the dishwasher almost every day, and they show very little wear, even after five years of daily use. Epicurean also makes gorgeous and easily washable silicone spatulas.

A sharp knife for chopping, coring and peeling is also helpful. Happy blending!

CHAPTER 4

January Smoothies

UNFILTERED APPLE JUICE SMOOTHIES

JANUARY 1: THE GOLDEN BANANA

Serves 2

Turmeric is a spice that adds a bright yellow color and a little bit of herbal flavor to this creamy banana-based, apple juice smoothie. Turmeric also helps balance the sweetness of the fruit flavors and aids in digestion.

Ingredients:

1 frozen banana

½ cup unfiltered apple juice

½ cup coconut water

½ cup ice

2 tablespoons hulled hemp seed

½ teaspoon lemon juice

½ teaspoon turmeric powder

Directions:

Combine all ingredients in a high-power blender
or food processor and blend until smooth.
Drink immediately.

Nutrition Facts (per serving):
Calories: 136 Fat: 3 Carbs: 25 Fiber: 3 Protein: 3

JANUARY 2: GINGER WARM-UP

Serves 2

The delicate apple and coconut flavors in this
smoothie get a zesty kick from ginger with a hot
bite from the fresh garlic.

Ingredients:

1 small garlic clove

½ cup coconut water

½ cup unfiltered apple juice

½ cup ice

2 tablespoons chia seed

1 teaspoon fresh ginger root

Directions:

Combine all ingredients in a high-power blender
or food processor and blend until smooth.
Drink immediately.

Nutrition Facts (per serving):
Calories: 111 Fat: 5 Carbs: 11 Fiber: 6 Protein: 3

JANUARY 3: GINGERED APPLE

Serves 1

This smoothie features a golden turmeric color, sweet
apple flavor and warm ginger undertones.

Ingredients:

½ cup unfiltered apple juice

½ cup ice

2 tablespoons chia seed

1 tablespoon fresh ginger root

½ teaspoon turmeric powder

1 pinch of ground cinnamon

Directions:

Combine all ingredients in a high-power blender or food processor and blend until smooth. Drink immediately.

Nutrition Facts (per serving):
Calories: 201 Fat: 10 Carbs: 17 Fiber: 12 Protein: 6

JANUARY 4: GINGERED APPLE MANGO

Serves 2

This smoothie is tropical and light with a little ginger heat! The mango contains digestive enzymes, which are soothing for many people who have digestive problems.

Ingredients:

½ cup unfiltered apple juice

½ cup mango

½ cup ice

2 tablespoons protein powder

1 teaspoon fresh ginger root

Directions:

Combine all ingredients in a high-power blender or food processor and blend until smooth. Drink immediately.

CULINARY TIP *Greek yogurt can be used in place of protein powder in any smoothie recipe, including this one.*

Nutrition Facts (per serving):
Calories: 76 Fat: 0 Carbs: 14 Fiber: 1 Protein: 5

JANUARY 5: APPLE GINGER LEMON

Serves 1

This smoothie provides a light blend with fresh ginger flavor and heat.

Ingredients:

½ cup unfiltered apple juice

½ cup ice

1 tablespoon fresh ginger root

1 tablespoon hulled hemp seed

2 teaspoons lemon juice

Directions:

Combine all ingredients in a high-power blender or food processor and blend until smooth. Drink immediately.

CULINARY TIP *If you're using a high-power blender, you should be able to simply remove the skin from the ginger root and let your blender do the rest of the work. Otherwise, you may need to chop your ginger root first before adding it to the blender.*

Nutrition Facts (per serving):
Calories: 106 Fat: 3 Carbs: 17 Fiber: 1 Protein: 3

JANUARY 6: SPICED APPLE

Serves 1

This cold refresher is aromatic, spicy and frosty. Cardamom seeds contain a range of essential oils that provide various medicinal effects, such as improving digestion.

Ingredients:

½ cup unfiltered apple juice

½ cup ice

1 tablespoon hulled hemp seed

1 teaspoon fresh ginger root

1 pinch of ground cardamom

1 pinch of ground cinnamon

Directions:

Combine all ingredients in a high-power blender or food processor and blend until smooth. Drink immediately.

CULINARY TIP *Add more ginger if you prefer more heat. You can also add up to 3 tablespoons of hulled hemp seed if you like the nutty flavor of hemp and want to boost protein.*

Nutrition Facts (per serving):
Calories: 103 Fat: 3 Carbs: 16 Fiber: 1 Protein: 3

JANUARY 7: GREEN TEA AND CHIA

Serves 2

This refreshing smoothie is like a slightly sweetened
iced tea. The apple juice and wild blueberries provide
the polyphenol antioxidant quercetin, which is
an anti-inflammatory.

Ingredients:

1 cup brewed green tea
½ cup frozen wild blueberries
½ cup unfiltered apple juice
½ cup ice
2 tablespoons chia seed

Directions:

Combine all ingredients in a high-power blender
or food processor and blend until smooth.
Drink immediately.

CULINARY **TIP** *Wild blueberries have a much
richer flavor than common
cultivated blueberries.*

Nutrition Facts (per serving):
Calories: 116 Fat: 5 Carbs: 13 Fiber: 8 Protein: 3

APPLESAUCE SMOOTHIES

JANUARY 8: APPLE BASIL BOOSTER

Serves 2

This smoothie provides a fresh apple flavor with the herbal scent of holy basil. A Harvard study found that those who eat anthocyanin rich foods, such as blueberries and apples, on a regular basis have a dramatically lower risk of type 2 diabetes.

Ingredients:

1 cup water

1 cup applesauce

½ cup ice

¼ cup fresh holy basil leaves

2 tablespoons chia seed

Directions:

Combine all ingredients in a high-power blender or food processor and blend until smooth. Drink immediately.

CULINARY TIP *Holy basil is an important herb in Ayurvedic medicine, as it supports blood sugar regulation. It is different from sweet basil and contains concentrations of nutrients that help boost our metabolism.*

Nutrition Facts (per serving):
Calories: 121 Fat: 5 Carbs: 15 Fiber: 7 Protein: 3

JANUARY 9: CHERRY GRAPEFRUIT VANILLA

Serves 2

This recipe is a play on the popular grapefruit-vanilla jelly doughnuts that are often available around the holidays. The turmeric powder used in this recipe is a powerful weight-loss aid, as it helps your body release stored water from body fat tissue.

Ingredients:

½ cup applesauce

½ cup frozen cherries

¼ cup grapefruit juice

2 tablespoons chia seed

1 teaspoon vanilla extract

¼ teaspoon turmeric powder

Directions:

Combine all ingredients in a high-power blender or food processor and blend until smooth.

Drink immediately.

Nutrition Facts (per serving):
Calories: 137 Fat: 5 Carbs: 17 Fiber: 8 Protein: 4

JANUARY 10: CHILLY CHERRY SLUSH

Serves 2

This smoothie has luscious, sweet apple and cherry flavors. It's perfect as a dessert after dinner to help improve your beauty sleep as the sweet cherries are a rich source of sleep-supporting melatonin.

Ingredients:

½ cup frozen sweet cherries

½ cup applesauce

½ cup coconut water

½ cup ice

2 tablespoons chia seed

Directions:

Combine all ingredients in a high-power blender or food processor and blend until smooth. Drink immediately.

 CULINARY TIP *Fruit sauces such as applesauce add enhanced flavor and an emulsifying ingredient.*

Nutrition Facts (per serving):
Calories: 130 Fat: 5 Carbs: 17 Fiber: 7 Protein: 4

HAZELNUT MILK SMOOTHIES

JANUARY 11: SPICED HAZELNUT APPLE

Serves 2

This delicious smoothie is dessert-like, fragrant and satisfying.

Ingredients:

½ vanilla bean

½ cup unfiltered apple juice

½ cup ice

½ cup hazelnut milk

2 tablespoons chia seed

1 pinch of ground cinnamon

Directions:

Combine all ingredients in a high-power blender
or food processor and blend until smooth.
Drink immediately.

Nutrition Facts (per serving):
Calories: 126 Fat: 6 Carbs: 13 Fiber: 6 Protein: 4

JANUARY 12: SWEET VANILLA HAZELNUT

Serves 1

This recipe is light, creamy and frosty with an essence
of vanilla. Vanilla extract is a flavoring that most of us
have in our kitchens and adds a lot of flavor without
adding sugar.

Ingredients:

1 Medjool date
½ cup hazelnut milk
½ cup ice
1 tablespoon protein powder
½ teaspoon vanilla extract

Directions:

Combine all ingredients in a high-power blender
or food processor and blend until smooth.
Drink immediately.

Nutrition Facts (per serving):
Calories: 149 Fat: 2 Carbs: 28 Fiber: 2 Protein: 6

JANUARY 13: HAZELNUT DATE SHAKE

Serves 1

The date used in this rich, creamy and slightly sweet shake contains fiber that slows the release of the date's natural sugar during metabolism. As a result, it has a low Glycemic Index even though it tastes very sweet.

Ingredients:

1 Medjool date

½ cup hazelnut milk

½ cup ice

1 tablespoon vanilla-flavored protein powder

Directions:

Combine all ingredients in a high-power blender or food processor and blend until smooth.
Drink immediately.

CULINARY TIP *Add up to 3 tablespoons of vanilla-flavored protein powder if you are drinking this smoothie as a meal replacement rather than a between-meal snack.*

Nutrition Facts (per serving):
Calories: 143 Fat: 2 Carbs: 28 Fiber: 2 Protein: 6

JANUARY 14: HAZELNUT CREAM FROSTY

Serves 2

This smoothie is creamy and rich with a light hazel-nut fragrance. The Greek yogurt used is strained and higher in protein than other types of yogurt. In fact, some Greek yogurt products are almost twice as high in protein.

Ingredients:

½ cup hazelnut milk

½ cup nonfat Greek yogurt

½ cup ice

1 tablespoon vanilla-flavored protein powder

1 teaspoon hazelnut extract

Directions:

Combine all ingredients in a high-power blender or food processor and blend until smooth. Drink immediately.

CULINARY TIP *Try out several different types of Greek yogurts to find the one that you like best. My favorite is FAGE Total 0% nonfat Greek yogurt, as it's mild and I love the creamy texture.*

Nutrition Facts (per serving):
Calories: 72 Fat: 1 Carbs: 7 Fiber: 0 Protein: 9

JANUARY 15: BERRY COBBLER

Serves 2

This recipe is basically a healthy wild berry cobbler in a glass with hints of lemon and vanilla. The wild blueberries in it provide anti-inflammatory polyphenols, and studies have shown that these polyphenols also improve cognitive function.

Ingredients:

1 Medjool date

½ cup hazelnut milk

½ cup ice

½ cup frozen wild blueberries

¼ cup gluten-free rolled oats

2 tablespoons chia seed

½ teaspoon vanilla extract

½ teaspoon lemon juice

Directions:

Combine all ingredients in a high-power blender or food processor and blend until smooth. Drink immediately.

CULINARY TIP

Cultivated or homegrown blueberries taste great in smoothies as well as wild blueberries.

Nutrition Facts (per serving):
Calories: 198 Fat: 7 Carbs: 28 Fiber: 10 Protein: 5

FRESH BANANA SMOOTHIES

JANUARY 16: PIÑA COLADA

Serves 2

This smoothie combines coconut, pineapple and banana in a creamy, sweet base.

Ingredients:

1 banana

1 cup coconut water

½ cup frozen pineapple

½ cup nonfat Greek yogurt

1 tablespoon unsweetened fine macaroon coconut

Directions:

Combine all ingredients in a high-power blender or food processor and blend until smooth.

Drink immediately.

Nutrition Facts (per serving):
Calories: 144 Fat: 2 Carbs: 27 Fiber: 3 Protein: 7

JANUARY 17: THE REVITALIZER

Serves 2

This smoothie is light and refreshing with a hint of vanilla. Think gelato with a perfect blend of sweet, cool and aromatic vanilla.

Ingredients:

½ banana

1 cup coconut water

½ cup nonfat Greek yogurt

½ cup ice

½ teaspoon vanilla extract

Directions:

Combine all ingredients in a high-power blender or food processor and blend until smooth. Drink immediately.

CULINARY TIP *Serve for dessert, as a palate cleanser between cheese appetizers or as an afternoon pick-me-up. To boost electrolytes after a night of drinking or a heavy workout, add a packet of electrolyte powder, such as Alacer's ElectroMix.*

Nutrition Facts (per serving):
Calories: 84 Fat: 0 Carbs: 15 Fiber: 1 Protein: 6

JANUARY 18: BANANA DATE

Serves 2

Greek yogurt and date sweeten this thick and spicy smoothie. Dates are a rich source of minerals and fiber, and they serve as a whole food sweetener for smoothies.

Ingredients:
1 Medjool date
½ banana
½ cup hemp milk
½ cup ice
½ cup nonfat Greek yogurt
1 teaspoon vanilla extract
¼ teaspoon cinnamon

Directions:

Combine all ingredients in a high-power blender or food processor and blend until smooth. Drink immediately.

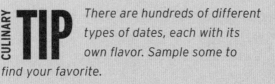

There are hundreds of different types of dates, each with its own flavor. Sample some to find your favorite.

Nutrition Facts (per serving):
Calories: 146 Fat: 1 Carbs: 24 Fiber: 2 Protein: 7

JANUARY 19: CHOCOLATE HAZELNUT MILK

Serves 1

This light and nutty smoothie is laced with vanilla and contains cocoa, a rich source of magnesium, which helps reduce cravings for sweets.

Ingredients:

½ banana

½ cup hazelnut milk

1 tablespoon unsweetened cocoa powder

1 tablespoon chia seed

½ teaspoon vanilla extract

Directions:

Combine all ingredients in a high-power blender or food processor and blend until smooth. Drink immediately.

Nutrition Facts (per serving):
Calories: 203 Fat: 8 Carbs: 26 Fiber: 9 Protein: 6

JANUARY 20: PB AND BANANA CREAM

Serves 1

Nuts and nut butters, such as peanut butter, provide protein and help to prevent dramatic carbohydrate-induced blood sugar spikes. This recipe has creamy banana with a little bit of the comforting peanut butter flavor.

Ingredients:

1 banana
½ cup oat milk
½ cup nonfat Greek yogurt
1 tablespoon peanut butter

Directions:

Combine all ingredients in a high-power blender or food processor and blend until smooth. Drink immediately.

CULINARY TIP *Because nut butters such as peanut butter add a lot of flavor, very little is needed.*

Nutrition Facts (per serving):
Calories: 331 Fat: 9 Carbs: 47 Fiber: 5 Protein: 20

JANUARY 21: APRÉS PLAY CAFÉ

Serves 1

Rehydrate yourself after playing hard and fuel up for more fun with this refreshing drink. In addition, the caffeine in coffee helps reduce inflammation triggered by intense athletic activity, which reduces pain.

Ingredients:

½ banana

½ cup coconut water

½ cup ice

1 tablespoon chia seed

1 teaspoon instant coffee

Directions:

Combine all ingredients in a high-power blender or food processor and blend until smooth. Drink immediately.

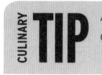 **CULINARY TIP** *Add 1 teaspoon of unsweetened cocoa powder for a mocha flavor.*

Nutrition Facts (per serving):
Calories: 143 Fat: 5 Carbs: 20 Fiber: 8 Protein: 4

JANUARY 22: COCONUT BANANA FIG

Serves 1

Banana carries the flavor in this sweet and creamy blend with hint of fig.

Ingredients:

1 fig

½ banana

½ cup coconut water

1 tablespoon chia seed

Directions:

Combine all ingredients in a high-power blender or food processor and blend until smooth. Drink immediately.

Nutrition Facts (per serving):
Calories: 180 Fat: 5 Carbs: 30 Fiber: 9 Protein: 4

JANUARY 23: MORNING ENERGY BOOST

Serves 2

This drink is creamy and easy on the palate first thing in the morning. In addition, whole grains such as those found in oatmeal appear to increase the production of cholecystokinin, a hormone involved in appetite control.

Ingredients:

1 banana

1 cup hemp milk

½ cup nonfat Greek yogurt

½ cup ice

¼ cup gluten-free oatmeal

1 teaspoon vanilla extract

1 pinch of ground cinnamon

Directions:

Combine all ingredients in a high-power blender or food processor and blend until smooth. Drink immediately.

CULINARY TIP *For more of a spice flavor, add more cinnamon to this blend.*

Nutrition Facts (per serving):
Calories: 209 Fat: 4 Carbs: 34 Fiber: 3 Protein: 10

JANUARY 24: HAZELNUT CREAM

Serves 2

This smoothie boasts strong hazelnut flavor in a creamy banana base. Bananas are a good source of the B vitamin folate, a key component for energy production.

Ingredients:

1 banana

½ cup hazelnut milk

½ cup ice

½ cup nonfat Greek yogurt

1 teaspoon hazelnut extract

1 teaspoon vanilla extract

Directions:

Combine all ingredients in a high-power blender or food processor and blend until smooth. Drink immediately.

Nutrition Facts (per serving):
Calories: 113 Fat: 1 Carbs: 21 Fiber: 2 Protein: 7

JANUARY 25: HAZELNUT LOVERS' DELIGHT

Serves 2

This recipe incorporates sweet hazelnut milk with a little banana flavor. Smoothies that contain more than 250 calories generally provide enough energy to be used as a meal replacement for breakfast to jump-start metabolism in the morning.

Ingredients:

1 banana

½ cup hazelnut milk

½ cup nonfat Greek yogurt

2 tablespoons chopped hazelnuts

1 teaspoon hazelnut extract

Directions:

Combine all ingredients in a high-power blender or food processor and blend until smooth. Drink immediately.

CULINARY TIP *Add up to an additional ¼ cup of chopped hazelnuts if you like a more crunchy texture in your smoothies.*

Nutrition Facts (per serving):
Calories: 291 Fat: 17 Carbs: 25 Fiber: 5 Protein: 11

JANUARY 26: CREAMY COCONUT PEACH

Serves 2

This delicious recipe has Hawaiian flavors with a peachy tartness.

Ingredients:

1 banana

½ cup frozen peach

½ cup coconut water

2 tablespoons chia seed

2 tablespoons unsweetened fine macaroon coconut

Directions:

Combine all ingredients in a high-power blender or food processor and blend until smooth. Drink immediately.

Nutrition Facts (per serving):
Calories: 164 Fat: 7 Carbs: 21 Fiber: 9 Protein: 4

JANUARY 27: CHOCOLATE FLIP

Serves 2

This drink is a lean chocolate dream. It's like drinking a chocolate sorbet, so drink it before it melts!

Ingredients:

1 banana
½ cup hemp milk
½ cup ice
½ cup nonfat Greek yogurt
2 tablespoons hulled hemp seed
1 tablespoon unsweetened cocoa powder
1 teaspoon vanilla extract

Directions:

Combine all ingredients in a high-power blender or food processor and blend until smooth. Drink immediately.

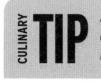 CULINARY **TIP** Add up to 3 tablespoons of cocoa powder to increase the chocolate factor.

Nutrition Facts (per serving):
Calories: 182 Fat: 5 Carbs: 24 Fiber: 3 Protein: 10

JANUARY 28: CHOCOLATE VANILLA SHAKE

Serves 2

Two all-American milkshake flavors—chocolate and vanilla—combine into one perfect smoothie!

Ingredients:

½ banana

1 cup hemp milk

½ cup nonfat Greek yogurt

2 teaspoons unsweetened cocoa powder

1 teaspoon vanilla extract

Directions:

Combine all ingredients in a high-power blender or food processor and blend until smooth. Drink immediately.

CULINARY TIP *Chocolate and vanilla are such popular flavors that this smoothie is the perfect combo for introducing smoothies to children or smoothie skeptics.*

Nutrition Facts (per serving):
Calories: 142 Fat: 3 Carbs: 20 Fiber: 2 Protein: 8

JANUARY 29: VANILLA THRILLA

Serves 2

This smoothie is simply comfort food in a glass.

Ingredients:

½ banana

½ cup oat milk

½ cup nonfat Greek yogurt

½ cup ice

½ teaspoon vanilla extract

Directions:

Combine all ingredients in a high-power blender
or food processor and blend until smooth.
Drink immediately.

CULINARY TIP *Skip the flavored yogurts, as they often contain high levels of sugar as well as synthetic coloring or flavors.*

Nutrition Facts (per serving):
Calories: 95 Fat: 1 Carbs: 15 Fiber: 1 Protein: 7

JANUARY 30: CHACE'S MORNING BOOST

Serves 1

This protein-rich smoothie is a simple daily breakfast
blend. Breakfast wakes up our metabolism and gives
us the energy and mental alertness we need to get our
day started right. It is my favorite blend. Hence the
name! When you don't have time to stop for lunch,
make yourself a "meal replacement" smoothie with
250-350 calories to keep you energized until dinner.

Ingredients:

1 banana
1 cup coconut water
½ cup nonfat Greek yogurt
½ cup frozen wild blueberries
1 tablespoon vanilla-flavored protein powder
½ teaspoon probiotics powder

Directions:

Combine all ingredients in a high-power blender
or food processor and blend until smooth.
Drink immediately.

Nutrition Facts (per serving):
Calories: 272 Fat: 1 Carbs: 53 Fiber: 6 Protein: 18

JANUARY 31: STRAWBERRY BANANA HEMP

Serves 2

This is a simple everyday smoothie that provides a metabolic boost in the morning.

Ingredients:

½ banana

1 cup organic hemp milk

½ cup frozen strawberries

2 tablespoons hulled hemp seed

Directions:

Combine all ingredients in a high-power blender or food processor and blend until smooth. Drink immediately.

CULINARY TIP *If you like a rich and creamy texture, then hemp milk is a good choice. If you prefer a lighter, frostier texture, then rice milk is a great liquid base.*

Nutrition Facts (per serving):
Calories: 154 Fat: 6 Carbs: 22 Fiber: 3 Protein: 4

CHAPTER 5

February Smoothies

CARROT JUICE SMOOTHIES

FEBRUARY 1: PEPPER CARROT

Serves 1

This smoothie is sweet and spicy with zing!

Ingredients:

½ cup carrot juice

½ cup ice

¼ cup medium-hot pepper

1 tablespoon chia seed

¼ teaspoon turmeric powder

Directions:

Combine all ingredients in a high-power blender or food processor and blend until smooth. Drink immediately.

Nutrition Facts (per serving):
Calories: 132 Fat: 5 Carbs: 15 Fiber: 8 Protein: 5

FEBRUARY 2: MIDWINTER HARVEST

Serves 2

This recipe is a fresh and delicious combination of carrot juice and fruit.

Ingredients:

½ apple
½ frozen banana
½ cup carrot juice
½ cup frozen strawberries
2 tablespoons chia seed
½ teaspoon lemon juice

Directions:

Combine all ingredients in a high-power blender or food processor and blend until smooth. Drink immediately.

Nutrition Facts (per serving):
Calories: 156 Fat: 5 Carbs: 23 Fiber: 9 Protein: 4

FEBRUARY 3: TOMATILLO CARROT

Serves 1

Carrot juice is a rich source of carotenoids, and this complex fruit and vegetable combination tastes like a fresh field of greens.

Ingredients:

2 tomatillos
1 cup carrot juice
½ cup ice
1 tablespoon chia seed
1 teaspoon lemon juice

Directions:

Combine all ingredients in a high-power blender
or food processor and blend until smooth.
Drink immediately.

CULINARY TIP Carrot juice is available in most
grocery stores these days, but
can also be made at home with
a juicer and stored in the fridge for up to a week
(see page 18).

Nutrition Facts (per serving):
Calories: 185 Fat: 6 Carbs: 27 Fiber: 9 Protein: 6

FEBRUARY 4: CARROT JUICE TISANE

Serves 1

This smoothie is slightly sweet, light and fortifying!

Ingredients:

1 cup brewed herbal tea
½ cup carrot juice
¼ cup ice
1 tablespoon chia seed

Directions:

Combine all ingredients in a high-power blender
or food processor and blend until smooth.
Drink immediately.

CULINARY TIP Add your favorite protein powder
or hemp seed to boost protein in
this simple smoothie. Herbal teas,
such as chamomile, blend well with carrot juice.

Nutrition Facts (per serving):
Calories: 117 Fat: 5 Carbs: 12 Fiber: 7 Protein: 4

FEBRUARY 5: WILD BLUE JUICE

Serves 1

This luscious smoothie is fragrant and earthy. Wild blueberries are preferable to common cultivated blueberries, as they have a richer flavor and twice the antioxidants. In addition, the hulled hemp seed used in the recipe provides omega-3 fatty acids that support weight loss in several ways, including by boosting mood and reducing cravings for fats.

Ingredients:

½ cup carrot juice
½ cup frozen wild blueberries
½ cup ice
2 tablespoons hulled hemp seed

Directions:

Combine all ingredients in a high-power blender or food processor and blend until smooth. Drink immediately.

CULINARY TIP *If you run out of carrot juice, unfiltered apple juice can be used instead, which tastes great in this combination.*

Nutrition Facts (per serving):
Calories: 172 Fat: 6 Carbs: 24 Fiber: 6 Protein: 6

FEBRUARY 6: BLOOD ORANGE FIZZ

Serves 2

This recipe is the perfect blend of fruit and vegetable. The blood orange's beautiful red pigment is from its anthocyanin antioxidants.

Ingredients:

1 blood orange

½ cup carrot juice

½ cup ice

2 tablespoons chia seed

½ cup sparkling water (such as San Pellegrino)

Directions:

Combine the blood orange, carrot juice, ice and chia seed in a high-power blender or food processor and blend until smooth. Then, stir in the sparkling water and drink immediately.

Nutrition Facts (per serving):
Calories: 127 Fat: 5 Carbs: 15 Fiber: 8 Protein: 4

FEBRUARY 7: MOJITO DIABLO

Serves 1

Studies of the Ayurvedic herb holy basil found that it helps lower blood sugar levels in people with type 2 diabetes. This mojito is sweet and crisp, with fresh basil and lime fragrance.

Ingredients:

½ cup carrot juice

½ cup fresh holy basil leaves

1 tablespoon lime juice

1 tablespoon chia seed

¼ teaspoon cayenne pepper

Directions:
Combine all ingredients in a high-power blender or food processor and blend until smooth. Drink immediately.

CULINARY TIP *Sweet carrots with hot pepper creates an ideal flavor combination.*

Nutrition Facts (per serving):
Calories: 119 Fat: 5 Carbs: 12 Fiber: 7 Protein: 5

FEBRUARY 8: GARLIC GINGER WARM-UP

Serves 2

This smoothie is a flavorful potpourri dominated by sweet carrots and spicy ginger. The holy basil used in this recipe has been proven in clinical studies to provide powerful anticancer benefits.

Ingredients:
1 garlic clove
½ cup carrot juice
½ cup ice
¼ cup fresh holy basil leaves
2 tablespoons fresh ginger root
2 tablespoons chia seed
1 teaspoon lemon juice

Directions:
Combine all ingredients in a high-power blender or food processor and blend until smooth. Drink immediately.

Nutrition Facts (per serving):
Calories: 100 Fat: 5 Carbs: 8 Fiber: 7 Protein: 4

FEBRUARY 9: HESTIA'S LOVE POTION

Serves 2

Tart cherries and fresh carrot juice give this smoothie a rich, sweet flavor. Tart cherries contain anthocyanins and salicylates that reduce inflammation and pain. I named this recipe for my friend Amy Boyer, who is known as Hestia, the Goddess of the hearth, because she creates beautiful homes for a living. This delicious combination not only reduces the aches and pains caused by physical work, but it also tastes amazing!

Ingredients:

1 cup frozen tart cherries
½ cup carrot juice
½ cup ice
2 tablespoons chia seed
1 teaspoon lemon juice

Directions:

Combine all ingredients in a high-power blender or food processor and blend until smooth.
Drink immediately.

Nutrition Facts (per serving):
Calories: 142 Fat: 5 Carbs: 19 Fiber: 8 Protein: 4

FEBRUARY 10: WINTER GREENS

Serves 2

This green drink has a rich carrot and pumpkin flavor.

Ingredients:

1 cup carrot juice

½ cup baby spinach leaves

½ cup ice

¼ cup canned pumpkin

2 tablespoons hulled hemp seed

½ teaspoon cinnamon

Directions:

Combine all ingredients in a high-power blender
or food processor and blend until smooth.
Drink immediately.

Nutrition Facts (per serving):
Calories: 103 Fat: 3 Carbs: 15 Fiber: 3 Protein: 4

FEBRUARY 11: TOMATILLO COOLER

Serves 2

Cilantro and lemon pair well in this carrot-
based smoothie.

Ingredients:

2 tomatillos

½ cup carrot juice

½ cup ice

¼ cup cilantro

2 tablespoons chia seed

1 tablespoon lemon juice

¼ teaspoon turmeric powder

1 pinch of fresh ground black pepper

Directions:

Combine all ingredients in a high-power blender or food processor and blend until smooth. Drink immediately.

Nutrition Facts (per serving):
Calories: 104 Fat: 5 Carbs: 9 Fiber: 7 Protein: 4

FEBRUARY 12: CARROT GINGER

Serves 1

This is the perfect veggie smoothie, as it is sweet, fresh and light. Additionally, a daily dose of fresh ginger root has been found to reduce muscle pain from exercise by 25%.

Ingredients:

½ cucumber

½ cup carrot juice

2 tablespoons fresh holy basil leaves

2 tablespoons cashews

1 teaspoon fresh ginger root

Directions:

Combine all ingredients in a high-power blender or food processor and blend until smooth. Drink immediately.

CULINARY TIP *A few drops of lemon juice can be added to brighten up this delectable combination.*

Nutrition Facts (per serving):
Calories: 218 Fat: 11 Carbs: 22 Fiber: 3 Protein: 7

FEBRUARY 13: THE HEALER

Serves 2

Sweet carrot juice balances the tannic greens and bitter turmeric in this healthy blend.

Ingredients:
½ frozen banana
1 cup carrot juice
½ cup fresh greens
½ cup nonfat Greek yogurt
½ teaspoon turmeric powder

Directions:
Combine all ingredients in a high-power blender or food processor and blend until smooth.
Drink immediately.

Nutrition Facts (per serving):
Calories: 108 Fat: 0 Carbs: 20 Fiber: 2 Protein: 8

HEMP MILK SMOOTHIES

FEBRUARY 14: HEMP POWER

Serves 1

This hemp combo is a delicious afternoon pick-me-up, as it provides omega-3 fatty acids and protein.

Ingredients:
1 cup hemp milk
½ cup ice
1 tablespoon hulled hemp seed
1 teaspoon vanilla extract

Directions:

Combine all ingredients in a high-power blender
or food processor and blend until smooth.
Drink immediately.

CULINARY TIP

Hemp is creamy but has very little
flavor. Punch up the flavor with
your favorite extracts such as
hazelnut, orange, almond or vanilla.

Nutrition Facts (per serving):
Calories: 197 Fat: 8 Carbs: 22 Fiber: 2 Protein: 6

FEBRUARY 15: HEMPBERRY SHAKE

Serves 2

This smoothie has a sweet berry flavor with a hint of
tart mango. The hemp milk provides a creamy texture
because it is rich in healthful essential fatty acids that
help us hydrate and reduce inflammation.

Ingredients:

1 cup hemp milk

½ cup frozen strawberries

¼ cup frozen mango

¼ cup ice

2 tablespoons chia seed

Directions:

Combine all ingredients in a high-power blender
or food processor and blend until smooth.
Drink immediately.

CULINARY TIP *This is a simple smoothie made from ingredients that can be stored in the refrigerator and freezer for months. The hemp milk comes in an aseptic package that has a long shelf life until opened.*

Nutrition Facts (per serving):
Calories: 165 Fat: 8 Carbs: 18 Fiber: 8 Protein: 5

FEBRUARY 16: THE ROSE THEATRE

Serves 2

Chocolate-covered dried cherries are a favorite snack at my beloved local movie theater in Port Townsend, Washington. This recipe is a smoothie version of this fabulous treat.

Ingredients:

½ frozen banana

½ cup hemp milk

½ cup ice

½ cup frozen cherries

2 tablespoons chia seed

1 tablespoon protein powder

1 tablespoon unsweetened cocoa powder

1 teaspoon vanilla extract

Directions:

Combine all ingredients in a high-power blender or food processor and blend until smooth.
Drink immediately.

Nutrition Facts (per serving):
Calories: 182 Fat: 7 Carbs: 20 Fiber: 8 Protein: 7

FEBRUARY 17: HEMP CHERRY CREAM

Serves 1

This classic comfort food smoothie is as thick and creamy as the milkshakes of my childhood.

Ingredients:

½ frozen banana

½ cup hemp milk

½ cup frozen cherries

1 tablespoon protein powder

Directions:

Combine all ingredients in a high-power blender or food processor and blend until smooth. Drink immediately.

CULINARY TIP *Hemp is one of the creamiest milk alternatives.*

Nutrition Facts (per serving):
Calories: 192 Fat: 3 Carbs: 36 Fiber: 4 Protein: 7

FEBRUARY 18: KIWI STRAWBERRY MILKSHAKE

Serves 2

This refreshing smoothie includes sweet strawberry and banana with a little bright, tart kiwi flavor. The antioxidants in kiwi can help reduce inflammation-induced arthritis pain when eaten daily.

Ingredients:

1 kiwi

½ frozen banana

1 cup hemp milk

½ cup frozen strawberries

2 tablespoons chia seed

Directions:

Combine all ingredients in a high-power blender
or food processor and blend until smooth.
Drink immediately.

CULINARY TIP *Fruit juice can replace the hemp milk in this recipe if you prefer a sweeter liquid to combine with the kiwi.*

Nutrition Facts (per serving):
Calories: 200 Fat: 8 Carbs: 26 Fiber: 9 Protein: 5

FEBRUARY 19: CREAMY MANGO

Serves 2

The fresh, sweet mango combined with the tangy
yogurt are a perfect combination in this carotenoid-
rich smoothie.

Ingredients:

1 cup mango

½ cup hemp milk

½ cup nonfat Greek yogurt

¼ cup ice

Directions:

Combine all ingredients in a high-power blender
or food processor and blend until smooth.
Drink immediately.

CULINARY TIP *Vanilla-flavored yogurt can be used to add another layer of flavor to this smoothie.*

Nutrition Facts (per serving):
Calories: 118 Fat: 2 Carbs: 20 Fiber: 2 Protein: 7

FEBRUARY 20: PEACHES AND CREAM

Serves 2

The plain yogurt used here generally has fewer calories and less sugar than flavored yogurt, such as vanilla, yet all the ingredients combine to create a sweet, creamy and light smoothie with a vanilla twist.

Ingredients:

1 frozen banana
1 peach
½ cup hemp milk
½ cup nonfat Greek yogurt
½ cup ice
1 teaspoon vanilla extract

Directions:

Combine all ingredients in a high-power blender or food processor and blend until smooth. Drink immediately.

CULINARY **TIP** *A vanilla bean in place of the vanilla extract adds more complex vanilla flavor and fragrance.*

Nutrition Facts (per serving):
Calories: 152 Fat: 1 Carbs: 27 Fiber: 3 Protein: 8

FEBRUARY 21: SWEET CREAM BREAKFAST SHAKE

Serves 2

The hemp milk used here helps make this smoothie creamy, sweet and rich in protein, whereas rice milk and nut milks generally don't contain protein.

Ingredients:

2 Medjool dates

½ cup hemp milk

½ cup nonfat Greek yogurt

½ cup ice

Directions:

Combine all ingredients in a high-power blender or food processor and blend until smooth. Drink immediately.

CULINARY TIP *Hemp milk gives smoothies a milkshake-like texture.*

Nutrition Facts (per serving):
Calories: 134 Fat: 1 Carbs: 25 Fiber: 2 Protein: 7

FEBRUARY 22: ICED COFFEE WHIP

Serves 1

This smoothie is similar to a decadent white frappe but full of protein. The instant coffee used in this recipe is just as effective as regular brewed coffee in decreasing the risk for type 2 diabetes.

Ingredients:

2 Medjool dates

½ cup hemp milk

½ cup ice

2 tablespoons protein powder

1 tablespoon instant coffee

Directions:

Combine all ingredients in a high-power blender or food processor and blend until smooth. Drink immediately.

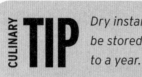

CULINARY TIP

Dry instant coffee granules can be stored in the freezer for up to a year.

Nutrition Facts (per serving):
Calories: 247 Fat: 3 Carbs: 47 Fiber: 4 Protein: 11

FEBRUARY 23: BANANA BASIL WHIP

Serves 2

This holy basil blend has subtle banana and hemp flavor. The hulled hemp seed not only tastes great but also provides gamma linolenic acid, which supports healthy hair, nails and skin.

Ingredients:
½ frozen banana
½ cup hemp milk
¼ cup fresh holy basil leaves
¼ cup ice
2 tablespoons hulled hemp seed

Directions:
Combine all ingredients in a high-power blender or food processor and blend until smooth. Drink immediately.

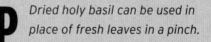

CULINARY TIP

Dried holy basil can be used in place of fresh leaves in a pinch.

Nutrition Facts (per serving):
Calories: 106 Fat: 4 Carbs: 13 Fiber: 2 Protein: 4

FEBRUARY 24: COFFEE AND CREAM

Serves 1

This blend tastes like cold and creamy vanilla coffee. Coffee inhibits free-radical damage to arterial linings, as it contains antioxidants, which reduce inflammation linked to heart disease.

Ingredients:

½ cup hemp milk
½ cup ice
½ cup nonfat Greek yogurt
1 tablespoon vanilla-flavored protein powder
1 tablespoon instant coffee

Directions:

Combine all ingredients in a high-power blender or food processor and blend until smooth. Drink immediately.

CULINARY TIP *Instant coffee is simply freeze-dried brewed coffee.*

Nutrition Facts (per serving):
Calories: 159 Fat: 3 Carbs: 15 Fiber: 1 Protein: 18

FEBRUARY 25: HEMP WHIP

Serves 2

Consuming 1 to 2 grams of whey protein per 2.2 pounds of body weight per day, in conjunction with strength training, may improve lean body mass. Try this creamy and light smoothie with a subtle vanilla flavor and a boost of whey protein.

Ingredients:

½ frozen banana

1 cup hemp milk

1 cup ice

2 tablespoons whey protein powder

1 teaspoon vanilla extract

Directions:

Combine all ingredients in a high-power blender
or food processor and blend until smooth.
Drink immediately.

CULINARY **TIP** *Whey protein powder dissolves well in smoothies and tastes delicious.*

Nutrition Facts (per serving):
Calories: 124 Fat: 3 Carbs: 18 Fiber: 1 Protein: 6

FEBRUARY 26: FIG COOKIE

Serves 2

This creamy hemp-based drink with almond and oat
nibbles is comfort food in a glass. It's also healthy, as
just three figs provide about 80 mg of calcium, which
helps us build muscles that burn extra calories.

Ingredients:

3 figs

½ cup hemp milk

½ cup ice

½ cup nonfat Greek yogurt

1 tablespoon roasted and chopped almonds

1 tablespoon gluten-free rolled oats

1 pinch of ground cinnamon

1 pinch of fresh ground nutmeg

Directions:

Combine all ingredients in a high-power blender or food processor and blend until smooth. Drink immediately.

Nutrition Facts (per serving):
Calories: 175 Fat: 5 Carbs: 25 Fiber: 4 Protein: 9

FEBRUARY 27: MOCHA MORNING BOOST

Serves 2

This is a classic high-protein mocha smoothie and a healthier morning frappuccino option rather than the high-fat, high-sugar, calorie-laden retail variety.

Ingredients:

½ frozen banana

1 cup hemp milk

½ cup ice

2 tablespoons chia seed

1 tablespoon instant coffee

1 tablespoon unsweetened cocoa powder

Directions:

Combine all ingredients in a high-power blender or food processor and blend until smooth. Drink immediately.

Nutrition Facts (per serving):
Calories: 176 Fat: 8 Carbs: 19 Fiber: 8 Protein: 5

FEBRUARY 28: CREAMY VANILLA PEAR

Serves 2

This smoothie combines light pear and vanilla flavors in a cream base.

Ingredients:

1 pear

½ cup hemp milk

½ cup nonfat Greek yogurt

½ cup ice

2 tablespoons vanilla-flavored protein powder

½ teaspoon vanilla extract

Directions:

Combine all ingredients in a high-power blender or food processor and blend until smooth. Drink immediately.

CULINARY TIP *Whey protein dissolves well and adds a creamy texture. If you are allergic to dairy, you may opt to skip the whey protein and try rice- or pea-based protein powders.*

Nutrition Facts (per serving):
Calories: 112 Fat: 0 Carbs: 17 Fiber: 2 Protein: 11

CHAPTER 6

March Smoothies

BLUEBERRY NECTAR SMOOTHIES

MARCH 1: BLUEBERRY VANILLA

Serves 2

This smoothie has rich blueberry flavor and just a hint of vanilla.

Ingredients:

½ cup frozen wild blueberries

½ cup blueberry nectar

½ cup ice

½ cup oat milk

2 tablespoons chia seed

½ teaspoon vanilla extract

Directions:

Combine all ingredients in a high-power blender or food processor and blend until smooth. Drink immediately.

CULINARY TIP *Wild blueberries are smaller, have a much stronger blueberry flavor and give more color to smoothies.*

Nutrition Facts (per serving):
Calories: 155 Fat: 6 Carbs: 20 Fiber: 8 Protein: 4

MARCH 2: VANILLA BERRY BANANA

Serves 2

The yogurt in this recipe gives this smoothie its creamy and thick texture.

Ingredients:

½ frozen banana

½ cup nonfat Greek yogurt

½ cup blueberry nectar

½ cup frozen strawberries

1 teaspoon vanilla extract

Directions:
Combine all ingredients in a high-power blender or food processor and blend until smooth. Drink immediately.

Nutrition Facts (per serving):
Calories: 111 Fat: 0 Carbs: 21 Fiber: 2 Protein: 6

MARCH 3: BERRY BLAST

Serves 2

This blend combines complex berry flavors in a light, frosty base. The blueberries and blackberries contain antioxidant anthocyanins that protect against memory loss.

Ingredients:

1 cup blueberry nectar

½ cup frozen wild blueberries

½ cup frozen wild blackberries

½ cup ice

2 tablespoons hulled hemp seed

Directions:

Combine all ingredients in a high-power blender or food processor and blend until smooth. Drink immediately.

CULINARY TIP

Add a teaspoon of honey to the smoothies if your berries are too tart.

Nutrition Facts (per serving):

Calories: 134 Fat: 2 Carbs: 27 Fiber: 4 Protein: 2

MARCH 4: PURPLE FAIRY

Serves 2

This elixir gives an intense blueberry flavor that is reminiscent of an afternoon in a berry patch.

Ingredients:

½ frozen banana

½ cup blueberry nectar

½ cup frozen wild blueberries

½ cup nonfat Greek yogurt

½ teaspoon vanilla extract

Directions:

Combine all ingredients in a high-power blender or food processor and blend until smooth. Drink immediately.

Nutrition Facts (per serving):
Calories: 112 Fat: 0 Carbs: 22 Fiber: 2 Protein: 6

MARCH 5: DOUBLE BLUEBERRY

Serves 2

Creamy with a gorgeous purple hue, this is a quick and easy everyday smoothie.

Ingredients:

½ cup frozen wild blueberries

½ cup blueberry nectar

½ cup ice

2 tablespoons vanilla-flavored protein powder

Directions:

Combine all ingredients in a high-power blender or food processor and blend until smooth. Drink immediately.

Nutrition Facts (per serving):
Calories: 71 Fat: 0 Carbs: 13 Fiber: 2 Protein: 4

MARCH 6: CREAMY VANILLA CHERRY

Serves 1

This delicious recipe is sweet and bright, and it has plenty of berry flavor. Heaven!

Ingredients:

½ cup blueberry nectar

½ cup cherries

1 tablespoon vanilla-flavored protein powder

Directions:

Combine all ingredients in a high-power blender or food processor and blend until smooth. Drink immediately.

Nutrition Facts (per serving):
Calories: 134 Fat: 0 Carbs: 29 Fiber: 2 Protein: 5

MARCH 7: BERRY MELON

Serves 2

This blend has a strong berry flavor with a little lemon twist.

Ingredients:

½ cup frozen blueberries

½ cup blueberry nectar

½ cup ice

½ cup honeydew melon

2 tablespoons chia seed

1 teaspoon lemon juice

Directions:

Combine all ingredients in a high-power blender or food processor and blend until smooth. Drink immediately.

Nutrition Facts (per serving):
Calories: 134 Fat: 5 Carbs: 17 Fiber: 8 Protein: 3

MARCH 8: GREEN BERRY

Serves 2

Enjoy your veggies in this antioxidant-rich,
date-sweetened, green drink.

Ingredients:

1 Medjool date
1 cup baby kale
½ cup blueberry nectar
½ cup ice
2 tablespoons chia seed

Directions:

Combine all ingredients in a high-power blender
or food processor and blend until smooth.
Drink immediately.

CULINARY TIP

*Kale is a brassica family vegetable
rich in beta-carotene, vitamin K,
vitamin C and calcium.*

Nutrition Facts (per serving):
Calories: 152 Fat: 5 Carbs: 21 Fiber: 7 Protein: 4

MARCH 9: BERRY MELON SLUSHY

Serves 1

Watermelon and blueberry are the perfect paring
in this delicious smoothie.

Ingredients:

1 cup watermelon
½ cup blueberry nectar
1 tablespoon protein powder
½ teaspoon lemon juice
¼ teaspoon vanilla extract

Directions:

Combine all ingredients in a high-power blender or food processor and blend until smooth. Drink immediately.

CULINARY TIP *Flavorings such as vanilla, orange or hazelnut extract add a sense of sweetness through flavor and scent without adding sugar. You can add up to 2 tablespoons of protein powder to boost the protein content.*

Nutrition Facts (per serving):
Calories: 135 Fat: 0 Carbs: 28 Fiber: 1 Protein: 5

FRESH HOLY BASIL LEAF SMOOTHIES

MARCH 10: HOLY BASIL ELIXIR

Serves 1

This is a simple and delicious blend of fresh herbs and apple flavor that is the perfect daily afternoon smoothie because of its medicinal support of weight loss.

Ingredients:

½ frozen banana

½ cup unfiltered apple juice

½ cup fresh holy basil leaves

1 tablespoon chia seed

Directions:

Combine all ingredients in a high-power blender or food processor and blend until smooth. Drink immediately.

CULINARY TIP *Add a cup of ice if you like your smoothies cold and slushy.*

Nutrition Facts (per serving):
Calories: 154 Fat: 5 Carbs: 22 Fiber: 7 Protein: 4

MARCH 11: CREAMY CHERRY FREEZE

Serves 2

In this creamy, tart cherry whip with a fresh herbal scent, coconut water provides the electrolytes that our muscles need to work properly.

Ingredients:

1 cup coconut water
½ cup ice
½ cup nonfat Greek yogurt
½ cup tart cherries
½ cup fresh holy basil leaves

Directions:

Combine all ingredients in a high-power blender or food processor and blend until smooth. Drink immediately.

CULINARY TIP *Fresh or frozen whole cherries provide so much tang that not much else is needed to flavor this smoothie for two.*

Nutrition Facts (per serving):
Calories: 74 Fat: 0 Carbs: 13 Fiber: 1 Protein: 6

MARCH 12: BASIL PEACH

Serves 2

Fresh holy basil leaves add fragrance and flavor to this peach and citrus smoothie.

Ingredients:

½ cup blueberry nectar

½ cup frozen peaches

½ cup ice

¼ cup fresh holy basil leaves

2 tablespoons chia seed

1 teaspoon lemon juice

Directions:

Combine all ingredients in a high-power blender or food processor and blend until smooth. Drink immediately.

Nutrition Facts (per serving):
Calories: 118 Fat: 5 Carbs: 13 Fiber: 7 Protein: 3

MARCH 13: CHOCOLATE ORANGE

Serves 1

This blended drink is a simple and delicious chocolaty-orange weight-loss formula.

Ingredients:

½ cup orange juice

½ cup ice

¼ cup fresh holy basil leaves

2 tablespoons chia seed

1 tablespoon unsweetened cocoa powder

Directions:

Combine all ingredients in a high-power blender or food processor and blend until smooth. Drink immediately.

Nutrition Facts (per serving):
Calories: 108 Fat: 6 Carbs: 9 Fiber: 7 Protein: 4

MARCH 14: GINGERED GRAPE

Serves 1

This smoothie tastes like a slushy grape soda with a little exotic ginger twist.

Ingredients:

½ cup grape juice

½ cup ice

¼ cup fresh holy basil leaves

1 tablespoon chia seed

1 teaspoon fresh ginger root

Directions:

Combine all ingredients in a high-power blender or food processor and blend until smooth. Drink immediately.

CULINARY TIP *Grape juice has such a strong, sweet flavor that a little goes a long way toward providing flavor without a lot of calories.*

Nutrition Facts (per serving):
Calories: 147 Fat: 5 Carbs: 20 Fiber: 6 Protein: 4

MARCH 15: BANANA BASIL

Serves 1

Enjoy the smooth coconut and banana flavors melded with fresh greens and a bit of herbal fragrance in this blend.

Ingredients:

½ frozen banana

½ cup coconut water

¼ cup fresh holy basil leaves

¼ cup spinach

2 tablespoons hulled hemp seed

Directions:

Combine all ingredients in a high-power blender or food processor and blend until smooth. Drink immediately.

Nutrition Facts (per serving):
Calories: 164 Fat: 6 Carbs: 22 Fiber: 4 Protein: 6

MARCH 16: SKINNY ELIXER

Serves 2

Rosmarinic acid is a natural phenolic in holy basil that supports metabolism, helps to reduce the development of body fat and eliminates extra water weight, making it an effective anti-inflammatory when taken daily.

Ingredients:

1 fig

½ cucumber

½ cup ice

½ cup unfiltered apple juice

¼ cup fresh holy basil leaves

¼ cup avocado

2 tablespoons chia seed

Directions:

Combine all ingredients in a high-power blender or food processor and blend until smooth. Drink immediately.

Nutrition Facts (per serving):
Calories: 158 Fat: 8 Carbs: 16 Fiber: 9 Protein: 4

MARCH 17: CARROT CANTALOUPE POWER ELIXIR

Serves 2

This elixir boasts a strange and wonderful combination with fresh scents, loads of protein and the weight-loss benefits of holy basil.

Ingredients:

1 cup carrot juice

1 cup frozen cantaloupe

½ cup nonfat Greek yogurt

¼ cup fresh holy basil leaves

2 tablespoons chia seed

Directions:

Combine all ingredients in a high-power blender or food processor and blend until smooth. Drink immediately.

Nutrition Facts (per serving):
Calories: 178 Fat: 5 Carbs: 21 Fiber: 8 Protein: 11

MARCH 18: PAPAYA LIME GINGER

Serves 1

This herbed papaya blend is mixed in a coconut base with a little ginger and lime.

Ingredients:

½ cup coconut water

½ cup frozen papaya

¼ cup fresh holy basil leaves

1 tablespoon chia seed

1 tablespoon fresh ginger root

½ teaspoon lime juice

Directions:

Combine all ingredients in a high-power blender
or food processor and blend until smooth.
Drink immediately.

Nutrition Facts (per serving):
Calories: 127 Fat: 5 Carbs: 16 Fiber: 7 Protein: 4

MARCH 19: SPICED CARROT

Serves 1

This recipe is a hot and spicy carrot puree.

Ingredients:

5 fresh holy basil leaves

½ cup carrot juice

½ cup ice

¼ cup medium-hot pepper

1 teaspoon fresh ginger root

1 pinch of fresh ground black pepper

1 pinch of cardamom

Directions:

Combine all ingredients in a high-power blender
or food processor and blend until smooth.
Drink immediately.

Nutrition Facts (per serving):
Calories: 63 Fat: 0 Carbs: 15 Fiber: 2 Protein: 2

OAT MILK SMOOTHIES

MARCH 20: SWEET DATE CREAM

Serves 1

This oat milk smoothie has a very comforting, soft flavor.

Ingredients:

1 Medjool date

½ cup oat milk

½ cup nonfat Greek yogurt

½ cup ice

1 pinch of fresh ground nutmeg

Directions:

Combine all ingredients in a high-power blender or food processor and blend until smooth. Drink immediately.

Nutrition Facts (per serving):
Calories: 189 Fat: 2 Carbs: 34 Fiber: 2 Protein: 14

MARCH 21: VANILLA BEAN BLIZZARD

Serves 2

This creamy, high-protein, frosty drink with rich vanilla flavor is a perfect dessert or bedtime snack to keep blood sugar levels from dropping low in the night.

Ingredients:

1 vanilla bean

1 cup oat milk

1 cup ice

1 cup nonfat Greek yogurt

½ teaspoon vanilla extract

Directions:
Combine all ingredients in a high-power blender
or food processor and blend until smooth.
Drink immediately.

Nutrition Facts (per serving):
Calories: 135 Fat: 1 Carbs: 17 Fiber: 1 Protein: 14

MARCH 22: CHERRY OAT BANANA

Serves 2

This smoothie combines creamy, rich banana with
sweet cherry goodness.

Ingredients:
1 frozen banana
½ cup oat milk
½ cup ice
½ cup frozen sweet cherries
2 tablespoons chia seed
½ teaspoon turmeric powder

Directions:
Combine all ingredients in a high-power blender
or food processor and blend until smooth.
Drink immediately.

Nutrition Facts (per serving):
Calories: 179 Fat: 6 Carbs: 27 Fiber: 9 Protein: 5

MARCH 23: SKINNY GRANOLA

Serves 2

This skinny smoothie is a low-fat blend of comforting flavors with just a hint of spice.

Ingredients:

1 frozen banana

½ cup oat milk

½ cup ice

2 tablespoons chia seed

1 tablespoon gluten-free oats

1 pinch of ground cinnamon

1 pinch of ground cardamom

Directions:

Combine all ingredients in a high-power blender or food processor and blend until smooth. Drink immediately.

Nutrition Facts (per serving):
Calories: 166 Fat: 6 Carbs: 22 Fiber: 8 Protein: 5

MARCH 24: CINNAMON PEAR

Serves 1

This smoothie has a mild, delicate flavor with just a hint of sweetness and spice.

Ingredients:

½ pear

½ cup oat milk

½ cup ice

1 tablespoon chia seed

Pinch of cinnamon

Directions:

Combine all ingredients in a high-power blender or food processor and blend until smooth.

Drink immediately.

CULINARY TIP *If you prefer more flavor intensity, add a pinch of nutmeg or fresh ground black pepper to spice it up.*

Nutrition Facts (per serving):
Calories: 186 Fat: 6 Carbs: 27 Fiber: 10 Protein: 5

MARCH 25: STRAWBERRY SHAKE

Serves 2

The sweet strawberries, creamy yogurt and scent of vanilla are comforting, and this smoothie is rich in protein and vitamin C.

Ingredients:

1 cup oat milk

1 cup frozen strawberries

½ cup nonfat Greek yogurt

½ cup ice

1 teaspoon vanilla extract

Directions:

Combine all ingredients in a high-power blender or food processor and blend until smooth.

Drink immediately.

Nutrition Facts (per serving):
Calories: 130 Fat: 1 Carbs: 21 Fiber: 3 Protein: 8

MARCH 26: CARDAMOM BANANA PEACH

Serves 2

This drink offers a taste of India in a glass. The cardamom provides exotic fragrance and flavor.

Ingredients:

1 frozen banana
1 frozen peach
½ cup oat milk
½ cup ice
½ cup nonfat Greek yogurt
1 tablespoon protein powder
½ teaspoon vanilla extract
½ teaspoon cardamom
¼ teaspoon cinnamon
1 pinch of fresh ground nutmeg

Directions:

Combine all ingredients in a high-power blender or food processor and blend until smooth. Drink immediately.

CULINARY TIP Ground nutmeg can be purchased, but the oils oxidize, leaving it bland. Therefore, to get the full nutmeg scent and flavor, keep whole nutmeg on hand and grate a little bit as needed.

Nutrition Facts (per serving):
Calories: 162 Fat: 1 Carbs: 30 Fiber: 3 Protein: 10

MARCH 27: PEACHES AND CREAM WITH BASIL

Serves 2

Holy basil adds a delicate herbal tone to this perfect pairing of oats and peaches. Holy basil also contains ursolic acid, which has been shown in laboratory studies to increase muscle and reduce body fat.

Ingredients:

1 cup frozen peaches

½ cup oat milk

½ cup ice

¼ cup fresh holy basil leaves

2 tablespoons chia seed

Directions:

Combine all ingredients in a high-power blender or food processor and blend until smooth. Drink immediately.

CULINARY TIP Add ½ a banana to sweeten this smoothie if your peaches are tart.

Nutrition Facts (per serving):
Calories: 133 Fat: 6 Carbs: 14 Fiber: 8 Protein: 5

MARCH 28: BEDTIME PINK DRINK

Serves 1

This balanced pink drink helps you wind down and enjoy a refreshing night's sleep. Start a new bedtime tradition!

Ingredients:

½ cup oat milk

½ cup frozen cherries

1 tablespoon protein powder

1 teaspoon powdered fiber supplement

Directions:

Combine all ingredients in a high-power blender or food processor and blend until smooth. Drink immediately.

CULINARY TIP *Fresh, raw cherries can be used in place of frozen cherries as long as they're pitted first.*

Nutrition Facts (per serving):
Calories: 145 Fat: 2 Carbs: 27 Fiber: 5 Protein: 7

MARCH 29: PB AND J

Serves 2

This drink has a classic peanut butter and jelly flavor and is packed with protein!

Ingredients:

1 cup oat milk

½ cup frozen strawberries

¼ cup gluten-free oats

2 tablespoons protein powder

1 tablespoon peanut butter

Directions:

Combine all ingredients in a high-power blender or food processor and blend until smooth. Drink immediately.

Nutrition Facts (per serving):
Calories: 195 Fat: 6 Carbs: 25 Fiber: 4 Protein: 10

MARCH 30: CHOCOLATE STRAWBERRY CREAM

Serves 2

This recipe is decadent, like chocolate-dipped strawberries, yet it helps you lose weight! Additionally, strawberries are a good source of fiber, which helps you reach the daily recommended intake of 25 to 30 grams.

Ingredients:

1 vanilla bean
½ cup oat milk
½ cup nonfat Greek yogurt
½ cup frozen strawberries
1 tablespoon unsweetened cocoa powder

Directions:

Combine all ingredients in a high-power blender or food processor and blend until smooth. Drink immediately.

CULINARY TIP *Whole vanilla beans can be ground up in high-power blenders. However, if your blender has a hard time with tough fibers, use vanilla extract or ground vanilla bean—otherwise, scrape out the seeds from inside of the vanilla beans, toss the husks and use the seeds in your smoothie.*

Nutrition Facts (per serving):
Calories: 89 Fat: 1 Carbs: 13 Fiber: 2 Protein: 8

MARCH 31: BERRY DELIGHT

Serves 2

The oat milk and Greek yogurt give this frosty blend a creamy base and the vanilla lends an amazing fragrance.

Ingredients:

½ cup frozen strawberries

½ cup oat milk

½ cup ice

½ cup nonfat Greek yogurt

½ teaspoon vanilla extract

Directions:

Combine all ingredients in a high-power blender or food processor and blend until smooth. Drink immediately.

CULINARY TIP *Buy organic strawberries for better flavor, increased nutrient levels and to avoid agricultural chemical residue.*

Nutrition Facts (per serving):
Calories: 82 Fat: 1 Carbs: 12 Fiber: 1 Protein: 8

CHAPTER 7

April Smoothies

PEAR SMOOTHIES

APRIL 1: VANILLA PEAR

Serves 1

Pear, lemon and vanilla are pure heaven in a glass!

Ingredients:

½ cup unfiltered apple juice

½ cup pear

½ cup ice

1 tablespoon chia seed

1 teaspoon lemon juice

½ teaspoon vanilla extract

Directions:

Combine all ingredients in a high-power blender
or food processor and blend until smooth.
Drink immediately.

Nutrition Facts (per serving):
Calories: 175 Fat: 5 Carbs: 27 Fiber: 9 Protein: 3

APRIL 2: VANILLA PEAR GINGER

Serves 1

Ginger heats up this pear blend.

Ingredients:

½ cup unfiltered apple juice

½ cup pear

½ cup ice

1 tablespoon chia seed

1 teaspoon fresh ginger root

½ teaspoon vanilla extract

Directions:

Combine all ingredients in a high-power blender or food processor and blend until smooth. Drink immediately.

Nutrition Facts (per serving):
Calories: 176 Fat: 5 Carbs: 27 Fiber: 9 Protein: 3

APRIL 3: EXOTIC ASIAN PEAR

Serves 2

This fat-melting combination has an exotic fragrance and complex flavors.

Ingredients:

1 Asian pear

½ cup unfiltered apple juice

½ cup ice

2 tablespoons chia seed

1 teaspoon fresh ginger root

1 teaspoon coconut nectar

½ teaspoon turmeric powder

½ teaspoon vanilla extract

1 pinch of fresh ground nutmeg

Directions:

Combine all ingredients in a high-power blender
or food processor and blend until smooth.
Drink immediately.

CULINARY TIP

*Add an apple instead of an Asian
pear for a little more intense
sweetness.*

Nutrition Facts (per serving):
Calories: 136 Fat: 5 Carbs: 17 Fiber: 8 Protein: 3

APRIL 4: VANILLA PEAR CREAM

Serves 2

You'll find a delicate flavor with a warm vanilla base
in this smoothie.

Ingredients:

1 Medjool date

½ pear

½ cup oat milk

½ cup ice

½ cup nonfat Greek yogurt

½ teaspoon vanilla extract

Directions:

Combine all ingredients in a high-power blender
or food processor and blend until smooth.
Drink immediately.

Nutrition Facts (per serving):
Calories: 127 Fat: 1 Carbs: 24 Fiber: 3 Protein: 7

GRAPEFRUIT JUICE SMOOTHIES

APRIL 5: GREEK BREAKFAST

Serves 1

This grapefruit juice cocktail includes tomato and fragrant basil.

Ingredients:

1 small tomato

½ cup carrot juice

½ cup grapefruit juice

½ cup nonfat Greek yogurt

¼ cup fresh holy basil leaves

Directions:

Combine all ingredients in a high-power blender or food processor and blend until smooth.

Drink immediately.

Nutrition Facts (per serving):

Calories: 176 Fat: 0 Carbs: 30 Fiber: 2 Protein: 14

APRIL 6: CITRUS CHILL

Serves 2

The chia seeds add protein to this citrusy smoothie, which supplies the amino acids we need for efficient weight loss.

Ingredients:

1 tangerine

½ cup grapefruit juice

½ cup tangerine juice

½ cup ice

2 tablespoons chia seed

Directions:

Combine all ingredients in a high-power blender or food processor and blend until smooth.
Drink immediately.

Nutrition Facts (per serving):
Calories: 139 Fat: 5 Carbs: 18 Fiber: 7 Protein: 4

APRIL 7: SWEET GRAPE AND SOUR LEMON

Serves 1

This smoothie is a sweet, little refreshing treat.

Ingredients:

½ cup grape juice

½ cup grapefruit juice

½ cup ice

2 tablespoons protein powder

1 tablespoon lemon juice

Directions:

Combine all ingredients in a high-power blender or food processor and blend until smooth.
Drink immediately.

Nutrition Facts (per serving):
Calories: 172 Fat: 0 Carbs: 32 Fiber: 0 Protein: 10

APRIL 8: SUNRISE

Serves 2

This tangy and sweet smoothie has rich cherry flavor.

Ingredients:

½ cup grapefruit juice

½ cup frozen wild blueberries

½ cup ice

¼ cup tart cherry juice

2 tablespoons chia seed

Directions:

Combine all ingredients in a high-power blender or food processor and blend until smooth. Drink immediately.

CULINARY TIP *Increase the tart cherry juice to a ½ cup for a deeper cherry flavor.*

Nutrition Facts (per serving):
Calories: 130 Fat: 5 Carbs: 16 Fiber: 8 Protein: 4

APRIL 9: THE GRAPEFRUIT REVITALIZER

Serves 2

This is a simple and quick smoothie to make when you're busy but need a little energy boost.

Ingredients:

1 banana

1 cup coconut water

½ cup grapefruit juice

½ cup ice

2 tablespoons protein powder

Directions:
Combine all ingredients in a high-power blender
or food processor and blend until smooth.
Drink immediately.

CULINARY TIP
*Adding a teaspoon of lemon juice
will add zing to this smoothie.*

Nutrition Facts (per serving):
Calories: 119 Fat: 0 Carbs: 25 Fiber: 2 Protein: 5

APRIL 10: GRAPEFRUIT ICY TEA

Serves 1

Grapefruit contains anti-inflammatory nutrients that
help us shed unwanted water weight when we eat
it on a regular basis. Enjoy the benefits in this light,
refreshing and slightly sweet treat.

Ingredients:
1 cup grapefruit
½ cup brewed green tea
¼ cup ice
1 tablespoon hulled hemp seed
1 teaspoon coconut nectar

Directions:
Combine all ingredients in a high-power blender
or food processor and blend until smooth.
Drink immediately.

CULINARY **TIP** *Add more hemp seed to increase the protein level of this drink, but be aware that too much hemp can add a bitterness to smoothies.*

Nutrition Facts (per serving):
Calories: 151 Fat: 3 Carbs: 30 Fiber: 5 Protein: 4

APRIL 11: GRAPEFRUIT AND GINGER

Serves 1

This drink is a citrus explosion with zingy ginger.

Ingredients:

½ cup tangerine juice

½ cup grapefruit

½ cup ice

2 tablespoons chia seed

1 teaspoon fresh ginger root

Directions:

Combine all ingredients in a high-power blender or food processor and blend until smooth. Drink immediately.

Nutrition Facts (per serving):
Calories: 262 Fat: 10 Carbs: 32 Fiber: 16 Protein: 8

GREEN SMOOTHIES

APRIL 12: GREEN AND CLEAN

Serves 1

Apple juice provides the base and greens provide the fresh-fields flavor in this recipe. Dark leafy greens are an excellent source of calcium. In fact, turnip greens provide 200 milligrams per cup.

Ingredients:

½ cup unfiltered apple juice

½ cup ice

¼ cup turnip greens

1 tablespoon chia seed

½ teaspoon lemon juice

Directions:

Combine all ingredients in a high-power blender or food processor and blend until smooth.

Drink immediately.

CULINARY TIP *If you don't have turnip greens, you can use any greens you happen to have on hand instead.*

Nutrition Facts (per serving):
Calories: 130 Fat: 4 Carbs: 21 Fiber: 6 Protein: 3

APRIL 13: FRESH GREENS

Serves 2

This smoothie is a simple and delicious blend of peach and orange flavors.

Ingredients:

½ cup nonfat Greek yogurt

½ cup frozen peaches

½ cup orange juice

½ cup greens

½ cup ice

Directions:

Combine all ingredients in a high-power blender or food processor and blend until smooth. Drink immediately.

CULINARY TIP *The sweet fruit flavors and rich texture balance the astringent nature of leafy greens well in this smoothie.*

Nutrition Facts (per serving):
Calories: 77 Fat: 0 Carbs: 13 Fiber: 1 Protein: 7

APRIL 14: GREEN APPLE BLUEBERRY

Serves 1

The wild blueberries used in this smoothie are rich in flavor and contain a higher concentration of antioxidants than cultivated blueberries.

Ingredients:

½ cup applesauce

½ cup baby spinach

½ cup frozen wild blueberries

¼ cup fresh holy basil leaves

1 tablespoon chia seed

1 teaspoon lemon juice

Directions:

Combine all ingredients in a high-power blender
or food processor and blend until smooth.
Drink immediately.

Nutrition Facts (per serving):
Calories: 79 Fat: 2 Carbs: 15 Fiber: 5 Protein: 2

APRIL 15: GREEN HULK

Serves 2

You won't taste the greens—you'll only taste the
tropical flavors—which makes this recipe a delicious
way to incorporate dark leafy greens, an excellent
non-dairy source of calcium, into your smoothie.

Ingredients:

½ frozen banana

½ cup unfiltered apple juice

½ cup ice

½ cup greens

2 tablespoons chia seed

1 tablespoon unsweetened fine macaroon coconut

Directions:

Combine all ingredients in a high-power blender
or food processor and blend until smooth.
Drink immediately.

Nutrition Facts (per serving):
Calories: 172 Fat: 9 Carbs: 22 Fiber: 8 Protein: 3

APRIL 16: BANANA CASHEW GREENS

Serves 1

This drink has delicious fresh banana and greens
with a hint of cinnamon.

Ingredients:

½ frozen banana

½ cup coconut water

¼ cup greens

2 tablespoons cashews

1 pinch of cinnamon

Directions:

Combine all ingredients in a high-power blender
or food processor and blend until smooth.
Drink immediately.

CULINARY TIP *Fresh young garden greens, such
as red chard, kale and spinach,
add delicate flavor to this smoothie.*

Nutrition Facts (per serving):
Calories: 172 Fat: 8 Carbs: 24 Fiber: 2 Protein: 4

APRIL 17: GINGER KALE

Serves 1

This green drink with warming ginger and a splash
of lime boosts weight loss. Additionally, the spinach
included in this recipe is a rich source of magnesium, which has been found to help ease migraine and
tension headaches.

Ingredients:

½ cup carrot juice

½ cup ice

½ cup kale

2 tablespoons chia seed

1 tablespoon fresh ginger root

1 teaspoon lime juice

Directions:

Combine all ingredients in a high-power blender
or food processor and blend until smooth.
Drink immediately.

Nutrition Facts (per serving):
Calories: 182 Fat: 10 Carbs: 11 Fiber: 13 Protein: 7

APRIL 18: GREEN BANANA SOOTHER

Serves 2

This soothing smoothie is creamy, sweet and green
with a fresh banana scent.

Ingredients:

2 Medjool dates

½ frozen banana

½ cup coconut water

½ cup ice

¼ cup greens

2 tablespoons vanilla-flavored protein powder

Directions:

Combine all ingredients in a high-power blender
or food processor and blend until smooth.
Drink immediately.

Nutrition Facts (per serving):
Calories: 125 Fat: 0 Carbs: 28 Fiber: 2 Protein: 5

TANGERINE JUICE SMOOTHIES

APRIL 19: CHOCOLATE KUMQUAT

Serves 2

This creamy smoothie has delicate citrus, coconut and cocoa flavors.

Ingredients:

3 kumquats

½ cup tangerine juice

½ cup coconut water

½ cup ice

½ cup nonfat Greek yogurt

1 tablespoon protein powder

1 teaspoon unsweetened cocoa powder

½ teaspoon vanilla extract

Directions:

Combine all ingredients in a high-power blender or food processor and blend until smooth. Drink immediately.

Nutrition Facts (per serving):
Calories: 107 Fat: 0 Carbs: 17 Fiber: 2 Protein: 9

APRIL 20: SOUR BERRY ICE

Serves 2

This icy blend is cool and refreshing with a hint of sour and sweet. The chia seed gives this smoothie body, and is rich in protein, essential fatty acids and fiber.

Ingredients:

½ cup coconut water

½ cup frozen raspberries

½ cup tangerine juice

½ cup ice

2 tablespoons chia seed

½ teaspoon turmeric powder

Directions:

Combine all ingredients in a high-power blender or food processor and blend until smooth. Drink immediately.

Nutrition Facts (per serving):
Calories: 122 Fat: 5 Carbs: 14 Fiber: 8 Protein: 4

APRIL 21: TANGERINE MINT COOLER

Serves 1

This smoothie is light, minty and slightly sweet. Drink this tangerine mint cooler in the morning to help rev up your metabolism.

Ingredients:

½ cup tangerine juice

½ cup ice

½ cup brewed green tea

¼ cup fresh mint leaves

2 tablespoons hulled hemp seed

Directions:

Combine all ingredients in a high-power blender or food processor and blend until smooth. Drink immediately.

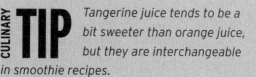

CULINARY TIP *Tangerine juice tends to be a bit sweeter than orange juice, but they are interchangeable in smoothie recipes.*

Nutrition Facts (per serving):
Calories: 147 Fat: 6 Carbs: 16 Fiber: 3 Protein: 6

APRIL 22: TROPICAL ENERGY BOOST

Serves 2

Enjoy this mango-banana boost with a little tangerine to sweeten. The hulled hemp seed included in this recipe is also nutritionally rich in protein and essential fatty acids.

Ingredients:

½ frozen banana

1 cup frozen mango

1 cup coconut water

¼ cup tangerine juice

2 tablespoons hulled hemp seed

Directions:

Combine all ingredients in a high-power blender or food processor and blend until smooth. Drink immediately.

CULINARY TIP *Hulled hemp seed is an ideal addition to smoothies because its flavor is neutral, it blends well and it comes in powder form.*

Nutrition Facts (per serving):
Calories: 155 Fat: 3 Carbs: 29 Fiber: 3 Protein: 4

APRIL 23: THE MAX GROVER

Serves 2

This weird, wonderful, heady and sweet drink is one of my favorite smoothies! The fresh pineapple used here is a rich source of antioxidants that help reduce inflammation.

Ingredients:

1 cup pineapple
½ cup tangerine juice
½ cup carrot juice
½ cup ice
2 tablespoons chia seed

Directions:

Combine all ingredients in a high-power blender or food processor and blend until smooth.
Drink immediately.

Nutrition Facts (per serving):
Calories: 161 Fat: 5 Carbs: 24 Fiber: 8 Protein: 4

APRIL 24: TANGERINE GINGER COCONUT

Serves 1

This recipe is sweet, gingery, light and fresh.

Ingredients:

½ cup coconut water
½ cup ice
½ cup non-fat Greek yogurt
¼ cup tangerine juice
1 tablespoon fresh ginger root

Directions:

Combine all ingredients in a high-power blender or food processor and blend until smooth. Drink immediately.

CULINARY **TIP** *Coconut water with ice is the perfect low-calorie, nutrient-rich smoothie base. Add your favorite fruit flavors and protein to create a personalized smoothie! And look for coconut water that has no added sugar.*

Nutrition Facts (per serving):
Calories: 118 Fat: 0 Carbs: 18 Fiber: 0 Protein: 12

APRIL 25: CHOCOLATE SUNRISE

Serves 1

This decadent smoothie is tart and sweet, like a cherry dipped in chocolate.

Ingredients:

½ cup tangerine juice

½ cup frozen wild blueberries

¼ cup black cherry juice

1 tablespoon chia seed

1 teaspoon unsweetened cocoa powder

Directions:

Combine all ingredients in a high-power blender or food processor and blend until smooth. Drink immediately.

CULINARY **TIP** *Add ice to give this smoothie a frostier texture.*

Nutrition Facts (per serving):
Calories: 196 Fat: 6 Carbs: 32 Fiber: 10 Protein: 4

APRIL 26: TART TANGERINE

Serves 1

This blended drink has a complex flavor without being too sweet.

Ingredients:

½ cup frozen peach
½ cup tangerine juice
½ cup ice
1 tablespoon chia seed

Directions:

Combine all ingredients in a high-power blender or food processor and blend until smooth. Drink immediately.

Nutrition Facts (per serving):
Calories: 153 Fat: 5 Carbs: 21 Fiber: 7 Protein: 4

APRIL 27: TANGERINE MELON MINT

Serves 2

The fresh mint leaf fragrance is beyond wonderful in this melon and citrus smoothie. Use brighter colored melons, such as cantaloupe, watermelon or crenshaw, to boost the skin-protecting carotenoids in this recipe.

Ingredients:

1 cup tangerine juice
½ cup honeydew melon
½ cup ice
¼ cup fresh mint leaves
2 tablespoons chia seed

Directions:

Combine all ingredients in a high-power blender or food processor and blend until smooth. Drink immediately.

Nutrition Facts (per serving):
Calories: 140 Fat: 5 Carbs: 18 Fiber: 7 Protein: 4

APRIL 28: GINGER CUCUMBER CITRUS

Serves 2

Tangerines give this smoothie a complex sweetness, and the ginger gives it a little heat. Additionally, the cucumber provides energy-enhancing electrolytes.

Ingredients:

½ cucumber

1 cup tangerine juice

½ cup ice

2 tablespoons chia seed

1 teaspoon fresh ginger root

1 teaspoon fresh lemon juice

Directions:

Combine all ingredients in a high-power blender or food processor and blend until smooth. Drink immediately.

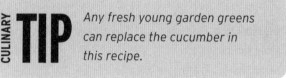

CULINARY TIP *Any fresh young garden greens can replace the cucumber in this recipe.*

Nutrition Facts (per serving):
Calories: 129 Fat: 5 Carbs: 15 Fiber: 7 Protein: 4

APRIL 29: MINT CUCUMBER CITRUS

Serves 2

Mint plays off the citrus in this fresh and
light smoothie.

Ingredients:

1 cup tangerine juice

½ cup cucumber

½ cup ice

¼ cup fresh mint leaves

¼ cup fresh holy basil leaves

2 tablespoons chia seed

Directions:

Combine all ingredients in a high-power blender
or food processor and blend until smooth.
Drink immediately.

 CULINARY TIP

*Ginger can be used instead of
mint to give this citrus smoothie
a flavor twist.*

Nutrition Facts (per serving):
Calories: 131 Fat: 5 Carbs: 15 Fiber: 7 Protein: 4

APRIL 30: HONEYDEW COOLER

Serves 2

This sweet and frosty drink also helps reduce inflammation.

Ingredients:

1 cup honeydew melon

1 cup ice

½ cup brewed green tea

¼ cup tangerine juice

2 tablespoons chia seed

½ teaspoon turmeric powder

Directions:

Combine all ingredients in a high-power blender or food processor and blend until smooth. Drink immediately.

Nutrition Facts (per serving):
Calories: 113 Fat: 5 Carbs: 12 Fiber: 7 Protein: 4

CHAPTER 8

May Smoothies

STRAWBERRY SMOOTHIES

MAY 1: WATERMELON STRAWBERRY

Serves 2

This light smoothie is packed with summertime-fresh strawberry flavor.

Ingredients:

1 cup watermelon

1 cup frozen strawberries

½ cup coconut water

2 tablespoons hulled hemp seed

Directions:

Combine all ingredients in a high-power blender or food processor and blend until smooth.
Drink immediately.

Nutrition Facts (per serving):
Calories: 104 Fat: 3 Carbs: 17 Fiber: 3 Protein: 3

MAY 2: STRAWBERRY BASIL ICY

Serves 2

This icy drink is aromatic and sweet with a light coconut flavor. The basil leaves contain an oil that is rich in antioxidants.

Ingredients:

1 cup coconut water
1 cup frozen strawberries
¼ cup fresh basil leaves
¼ cup ice
2 tablespoons chia seed

Directions:

Combine all ingredients in a high-power blender or food processor and blend until smooth. Drink immediately.

CULINARY TIP *Fresh basil can be found in most grocery stores or can be grown in your own home herb garden.*

Nutrition Facts (per serving):
Calories: 118 Fat: 5 Carbs: 13 Fiber: 8 Protein: 3

MAY 3: STRAWBERRY COOLER

Serves 2

This refreshing, sweet and spicy version of lemonade includes ginger, a mild anti-inflammatory.

Ingredients:

1 cup frozen strawberries
1 cup coconut water
2 tablespoons chia seed

1 teaspoon fresh ginger root

1 teaspoon lemon juice

1 cup sparkling water

Directions:

Combine strawberries, coconut water, chia seed, ginger and lemon juice in a blender or food processor and blend until smooth. Then, stir in the sparkling water and drink immediately.

CULINARY TIP *Use lime juice if you don't have lemon juice or if you prefer the lime flavor. Lemon or lime segments can also be used in place of juice.*

Nutrition Facts (per serving):
Calories: 118 Fat: 5 Carbs: 13 Fiber: 8 Protein: 3

MAY 4: STRAWBERRY MINT

Serves 2

This smoothie is thick and frosty with a light mint fragrance, and it's low in calories and contains no fat.

Ingredients:

½ cup coconut water

½ cup frozen strawberries

1 tablespoon protein powder

1 tablespoon fresh mint leaves

Directions:

Combine all ingredients in a high-power blender or food processor and blend until smooth.
Drink immediately.

Nutrition Facts (per serving):
Calories: 69 Fat: 0 Carbs: 13 Fiber: 2 Protein: 5

MAY 5: STRAWBERRY VANILLA POWER

Serves 1

This strawberry smoothie has intense vanilla undertones.

Ingredients:

1 cup frozen strawberries

½ cup rice milk

2 tablespoons protein powder

1 teaspoon vanilla extract

Directions:

Combine all ingredients in a high-power blender or food processor and blend until smooth. Drink immediately.

 CULINARY TIP *Try a vanilla bean rather than vanilla extract for an even more intense vanilla flavor.*

Nutrition Facts (per serving):
Calories: 169 Fat: 2 Carbs: 27 Fiber: 3 Protein: 10

MAY 6: RED, WHITE AND BLUE

Serves 2

Strawberries contain phenolic compounds that boost immune functions and support metabolic health.

Ingredients:

½ cup frozen strawberries

½ cup frozen blueberries

½ cup rice milk

½ cup ice

2 tablespoons chia seed

Directions:

Combine all ingredients in a high-power blender or food processor and blend until smooth. Drink immediately.

Nutrition Facts (per serving):
Calories: 130 Fat: 6 Carbs: 15 Fiber: 8 Protein: 3

MAY 7: ORANGE CHERRY STRAWBERRY

Serves 2

This frosty, sweet blend includes fresh berry and citrus flavors.

Ingredients:

1 navel orange

½ cup frozen strawberries

½ cup coconut water

½ cup frozen cherries

2 tablespoons chia seed

Directions:

Combine all ingredients in a high-power blender or food processor and blend until smooth. Drink immediately.

Nutrition Facts (per serving):
Calories: 151 Fat: 5 Carbs: 22 Fiber: 9 Protein: 4

MAY 8: GINGER BERRY SPICE

Serves 2

This smoothie has a rich berry flavor with a bouquet of ginger and spice. Additionally, piperine, the active ingredient in black pepper, may boost turmeric's anti-inflammatory action by 2000% by increasing the bio-availability of curcumin.

Ingredients:

½ cup blackberries

½ cup frozen strawberries

½ cup ice

¼ cup coconut water

2 tablespoons chia seed

½ teaspoon fresh ginger root

½ teaspoon turmeric powder

1 pinch of fresh ground black pepper

Directions:

Combine all ingredients in a high-power blender
or food processor and blend until smooth.
Drink immediately.

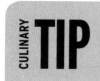

CULINARY **TIP** *Add more coconut water if more
liquid is needed to blend properly.*

Nutrition Facts (per serving):
Calories: 112 Fat: 5 Carbs: 12 Fiber: 9 Protein: 4

MAY 9: CHERRY BERRY PEACH

Serves 2

This frosty blend of fresh fruit flavors includes hemp
protein and a little citrus.

Ingredients:

1 cup cherries

½ cup coconut water

½ cup frozen peaches

½ cup frozen strawberries

2 tablespoons hulled hemp seed

1 teaspoon lemon juice

Directions:

Combine all ingredients in a high-power blender or food processor and blend until smooth. Drink immediately.

....

Nutrition Facts (per serving):
Calories: 132 Fat: 3 Carbs: 24 Fiber: 4 Protein: 4

MAY 10: BERRY POM PEACH

Serves 2

....

This sweet and sour drink is rich in fruit flavors and a delicious way to wake up and start your day! Punicalagins are the acidic tannins in pomegranate that provide free radical–scavenging health properties.

....

Ingredients:

1 cup coconut water

½ cup ice

¼ cup frozen wild blueberries

¼ cup pomegranate juice

¼ cup frozen strawberries

¼ cup frozen peaches

2 tablespoons hulled hemp seed

....

Directions:

Combine all ingredients in a high-power blender or food processor and blend until smooth. Drink immediately.

CULINARY TIP *Pomegranate juice is a rich source of antioxidants, but it can be a bit sour. The fruity combination in this smoothie helps sweeten and soften the intensity of the acidic tannins in the pomegranate.*

Nutrition Facts (per serving):
Calories: 111 Fat: 6 Carbs: 34 Fiber: 5 Protein: 6

CANTALOUPE SMOOTHIES

MAY 11: CANTALOUPE CITRUS TWIST

Serves 2

This fresh smoothie gets its sweet apple flavor from the apple and the unfiltered apple juice, which contains more of the apple's natural fiber than clear apple juice.

Ingredients:

½ apple

1 cup cantaloupe

½ cup unfiltered apple juice

½ cup ice

2 tablespoons chia seed

1 tablespoon lemon juice

Directions:

Combine all ingredients in a high-power blender or food processor and blend until smooth. Drink immediately.

Nutrition Facts (per serving):
Calories: 149 Fat: 5 Carbs: 21 Fiber: 8 Protein: 4

MAY 12: CREAMY MELON

Serves 2

This smoothie is a blend of intricate flavors, as prunes add a bit of sweetness and fragrance and the cantaloupe adds a fresh scent.

Ingredients:

2 prunes

½ cup hemp milk

½ cup cantaloupe

½ cup nonfat Greek yogurt

¼ cup ice

Directions:

Combine all ingredients in a high-power blender
or food processor and blend until smooth.
Drink immediately.

Nutrition Facts (per serving):
Calories: 104 Fat: 1 Carbs: 17 Fiber: 1 Protein: 7

MAY 13: BERRY MELON PUNCH

Serves 2

This strawberry and melon combination has a trace
of ginger and coconut flavors. The hemp seed is an
excellent vegan source of protein.

Ingredients:

1 cup coconut water

1 cup frozen strawberries

1 cup cantaloupe

2 tablespoons hulled hemp seed

1 teaspoon fresh ginger root

Directions:

Combine all ingredients in a high-power blender
or food processor and blend until smooth.
Drink immediately.

Nutrition Facts (per serving):
Calories: 120 Fat: 3 Carbs: 21 Fiber: 3 Protein: 4

FRESH MINT SMOOTHIES

MAY 14: MINT TEA SLUSHY

Serves 2

This combination has subtle tea and mint undertones. According to recent studies, just one to two cups of green tea per day is ideal for fostering weight loss.

Ingredients:

½ cucumber

1 cup brewed green tea

1 cup frozen cantaloupe

½ cup ice

½ cup fresh mint leaves

2 tablespoons chia seed

Directions:

Combine all ingredients in a high-power blender or food processor and blend until smooth. Drink immediately.

CULINARY TIP *Brew green tea for no longer than 2 minutes, as this allows for the maximum nutrient infusion into the tea water without the bitter elements.*

Nutrition Facts (per serving):
Calories: 107 Fat: 5 Carbs: 10 Fiber: 8 Protein: 4

MAY 15: CUCUMBER MINT

Serves 2

This melon and cucumber drink has just a hint of mint, and the hemp seed is rich in inflammation-reducing omega-3 fatty acids.

Ingredients:

½ cucumber

1 cup coconut water

1 cup honeydew melon

½ cup ice

½ cup fresh mint leaves

2 tablespoons hulled hemp seed

Directions:

Combine all ingredients in a high-power blender or food processor and blend until smooth. Drink immediately.

CULINARY TIP *Hemp seeds taste like sesame seeds, but they're softer and blend well into smoothies.*

Nutrition Facts (per serving):
Calories: 107 Fat: 3 Carbs: 17 Fiber: 3 Protein: 4

MAY 16: BERRIES AND CREAM

Serves 2

Enjoy the hint of mint in this creamy strawberry shake.

Ingredients:

1 cup frozen strawberries

½ cup coconut water

½ cup nonfat Greek yogurt

½ cup ice

2 tablespoons protein powder

1 tablespoon fresh mint leaves

Directions:

Combine all ingredients in a high-power blender or food processor and blend until smooth. Drink immediately.

Nutrition Facts (per serving):
Calories: 93 Fat: 0 Carbs: 13 Fiber: 2 Protein: 11

MAY 17: BLACKBERRY JULEP

Serves 2

The wild blackberries in this smoothie give it a thick, sweet and satisfying flavor, and they provide concentrated levels of polyphenols.

Ingredients:

1 cup frozen wild blackberries

½ cup ice

½ cup water

¼ cup fresh mint leaves

2 tablespoons chia seed

Directions:

Combine all ingredients in a high-power blender or food processor and blend until smooth. Drink immediately.

CULINARY TIP

You can sweeten this shake even more by adding 1 to 2 dates or prunes.

Nutrition Facts (per serving):
Calories: 131 Fat: 5 Carbs: 13 Fiber: 10 Protein: 4

MAY 18: MINT APPLE POM

Serves 1

Apple juice takes the tartness out of the pomegranate, and the mint gives this smoothie a wonderful scent.

Ingredients:
½ cup unfiltered apple juice
½ cup ice
¼ cup pomegranate juice
2 tablespoons chia seed
1 tablespoon fresh mint leaves

Directions:
Combine all ingredients in a high-power blender or food processor and blend until smooth.
Drink immediately.

Nutrition Facts (per serving):
Calories: 230 Fat: 10 Carbs: 24 Fiber: 12 Protein: 6

MAY 19: APPLE MINT APERITIF

Serves 2

The fresh mint fragrance hits the nose before the sweetness and mint and lemon flavors hit the palate in this healthful shake.

Ingredients:
½ Fuji apple
½ cup unfiltered apple juice
½ cup ice
¼ cup fresh mint leaves
2 tablespoons chia seed
½ teaspoon lemon juice

Directions:

Combine all ingredients in a high-power blender
or food processor and blend until smooth.
Drink immediately.

....

Nutrition Facts (per serving):
Calories: 124 Fat: 5 Carbs: 15 Fiber: 7 Protein: 3

MAY 20: MINT LEMONADE REFRESHER

Serves 1

....

The fresh apple flavor with a hint of mint and citrus is
a hydrating combination perfect for the late afternoon,
when we're most dehydrated and tired from a busy day.

....

Ingredients:

½ cup unfiltered apple juice

½ cup ice

¼ cup fresh mint leaves

1 tablespoon lemon juice

1 tablespoon hulled hemp seed

....

Directions:

Combine all ingredients in a high-power blender
or food processor and blend until smooth.
Drink immediately.

CULINARY TIP *There are many types of mint, each with its own particular flavor. Taste your mint before adding it to your smoothie to make sure you like the flavor and so you can adjust the amount depending on its level of intensity.*

Nutrition Facts (per serving):
Calories: 106 Fat: 3 Carbs: 16 Fiber: 2 Protein: 3

MAY 21: MANGO MINT WITH CITRUS

Serves 1

This smoothie contains quercetin, an antioxidant flavonoid found in apples, which is a powerful anti-inflammatory and important for those with inflammatory conditions, such as food allergies, arthritis and cancer.

Ingredients:

5 fresh mint leaves

½ cup unfiltered apple juice

½ cup frozen mango

½ cup nonfat Greek yogurt

1 tablespoon lemon juice

1 teaspoon fresh ginger root

Directions:

Combine all ingredients in a high-power blender or food processor and blend until smooth. Drink immediately.

CULINARY TIP *In any smoothie recipe, you can use either fresh lemon juice or bottled lemon juice, which is easier to keep on hand and tastes just as good.*

Nutrition Facts (per serving):
Calories: 87 Fat: 0 Carbs: 16 Fiber: 1 Protein: 6

MAY 22: SAVORY SUMMER MIX

Serves 2

This combination includes cool green veggies with a minty scent. The greens are not only earthy and flavorful, but they also provide concentrated nutrients. A ½ cup of kale contains 45 milligrams of calcium, which promotes weight loss by increasing muscle activity, thereby increasing calories burned.

Ingredients:

1 tomato
½ cup fresh mint leaves
½ cup baby kale leaves
½ cup ice
2 tablespoons chia seed

Directions:

Combine all ingredients in a high-power blender or food processor and blend until smooth.
Drink immediately.

Nutrition Facts (per serving):
Calories: 93 Fat: 5 Carbs: 6 Fiber: 8 Protein: 4

NECTARINE SMOOTHIES

MAY 23: CHERRY ALMOND NECTARINE

Serves 2

Enjoy this nectarine and almond frosty with sweet cherries, which provide more carotenoids than most berries and stone fruits.

Ingredients:

1 nectarine

½ cup almond milk

½ cup ice

½ cup frozen sweet cherries

2 tablespoons hulled hemp seed

Directions:

Combine all ingredients in a high-power blender or food processor and blend until smooth. Drink immediately.

Nutrition Facts (per serving):
Calories: 104 Fat: 4 Carbs: 14 Fiber: 3 Protein: 4

MAY 24: NECTARINE AND MANGO

Serves 2

This smoothie is like a sorbet with rich, fruity flavors. The mango is rich in prebiotic dietary fiber that improves our metabolism by activating the beneficial bacteria in our digestive system.

Ingredients:

2 nectarines

½ cup cultured coconut milk

½ cup frozen mango

2 tablespoons chia seed

Directions:

Combine all ingredients in a high-power blender
or food processor and blend until smooth.
Drink immediately.

CULINARY **TIP** *Unripe nectarines can be a bit sour,
in which case adding a ½ teaspoon
of honey or coconut nectar will
perfect this recipe.*

Nutrition Facts (per serving):
Calories: 168 Fat: 7 Carbs: 22 Fiber: 10 Protein: 5

MAY 25: NECTARINE AND KIWI

Serves 2

This smoothie is tart and tangy and tastes
like summer!

Ingredients:

2 nectarines

1 kiwi

½ cup coconut water

½ cup ice

2 tablespoons chia seed

Directions:

Combine all ingredients in a high-power blender
or food processor and blend until smooth.
Drink immediately.

Nutrition Facts (per serving):
Calories: 158 Fat: 5 Carbs: 22 Fiber: 9 Protein: 5

FRESH PINEAPPLE SMOOTHIES

MAY 26: THE PURPLE MERMAID

Serves 2

This smoothie has tropical flavors with a citrus twist. The coconut water is an excellent source of electrolytes, which conduct electrical impulses throughout our bodies, keeping our energy systems at peak performance.

Ingredients:

1 cup pineapple

1 cup coconut water

½ cup frozen wild blueberries

2 tablespoons chia seed

½ teaspoon lemon juice

Directions:

Combine all ingredients in a high-power blender or food processor and blend until smooth. Drink immediately.

CULINARY TIP *If you mix any sweet fruit with coconut water and wild blueberries, chances are the result is going to be delicious.*

Nutrition Facts (per serving):
Calories: 150 Fat: 5 Carbs: 22 Fiber: 9 Protein: 3

MAY 27: RUBY SUNRISE

Serves 2

This sweet, fresh combination has a light citrus flavor and fragrance. The pineapple contains the digestive enzyme bromelain, which breaks down protein.

Ingredients:

1 cup water

½ cup frozen strawberries

½ cup pineapple

¼ cup ice

1 tablespoon hulled hemp seed

1 teaspoon Meyer lemon juice

Directions:

Combine all ingredients in a high-power blender or food processor and blend until smooth. Drink immediately.

CULINARY TIP *Meyer lemon juice is slightly sweeter and more fragrant than most lemons and lemon juices, so it's a favorite; however, any type of lemon juice works well in this recipe.*

Nutrition Facts (per serving):
Calories: 56 Fat: 2 Carbs: 10 Fiber: 2 Protein: 2

MAY 28: PINEAPPLE POM

Serves 2

This cocktail is sweet and tart with a light coconut taste. Polyphenols in the pomegranate seed helps reduce inflammation by disrupting the inflammatory signaling pathways.

Ingredients:

1 cup coconut water

½ cup ice

½ cup pineapple

¼ cup pomegranate seed

2 tablespoons chia seed

Directions:

Combine all ingredients in a high-power blender
or food processor and blend until smooth.
Drink immediately.

CULINARY **TIP** *The sweet intensity of pineapple is the perfect pairing with the tartness of the pomegranate seed.*

Nutrition Facts (per serving):
Calories: 130 Fat: 5 Carbs: 16 Fiber: 7 Protein: 4

MAY 29: SWEET PINEAPPLE GREENS

Serves 2

This green smoothie is sweet enough for kids!

Ingredients:

½ frozen banana

½ cup almond milk

½ cup pineapple

¼ cup baby spinach leaves

2 tablespoons chia seed

Directions:

Combine all ingredients in a high-power blender
or food processor and blend until smooth.
Drink immediately.

CULINARY TIP *Pineapple helps sweeten the spinach in this green drink.*

Nutrition Facts (per serving):
Calories: 124 Fat: 6 Carbs: 13 Fiber: 7 Protein: 4

MAY 30: ORANGE PINEAPPLE VANILLA

Serves 2

This smoothie is the perfect blend of citrus, tropical fragrance and vanilla. Studies have found that the scent of vanilla can help to reduce anxiety.

Ingredients:

½ cup orange juice

½ cup ice

½ cup pineapple

½ cup nonfat Greek yogurt

1 teaspoon vanilla extract

Directions:

Combine all ingredients in a high-power blender or food processor and blend until smooth.

Drink immediately.

CULINARY TIP *Plain yogurt has no added sugar, but flavored versions often pack in the sugar. Add your own vanilla flavor extract or a vanilla bean to plain yogurt to enjoy all the flavor without the added sugar and calories.*

Nutrition Facts (per serving):
Calories: 87 Fat: 0 Carbs: 14 Fiber: 1 Protein: 7

MAY 31: MINT MANGO DREAM

Serves 2

This mango and papaya nectar blend is thick and fresh with a bit of balmy mint. Cryptoxanthin, a carotenoid found in papaya, helps protect the skin from potential carcinogens, such as ultraviolet radiation from the sun.

Ingredients:

½ cup mango

½ cup papaya nectar

½ cup pineapple

¼ cup fresh mint leaves

¼ cup fresh holy basil leaves

2 tablespoons chia seed

Directions:

Combine all ingredients in a high-power blender or food processor and blend until smooth. Drink immediately.

CULINARY TIP *You can use frozen mango and pineapple if desired, but then increase the fruit juice (papaya nectar) to 1 cup.*

Nutrition Facts (per serving):
Calories: 150 Fat: 5 Carbs: 21 Fiber: 8 Protein: 4

CHAPTER 9

June Smoothies

APRICOT NECTAR SMOOTHIES

JUNE 1: APRICOT POWER BREAKFAST

Serves 1

This refreshing elixir has a sweet and aromatic apricot flavor with a frosty, creamy base. The probiotics included here help us drop weight by improving our digestion and metabolism.

Ingredients:

½ cup apricot nectar

½ cup ice

½ cup nonfat Greek yogurt

1 tablespoon protein powder

¼ teaspoon probiotic supplement

Directions:

Combine all ingredients in a high-power blender or food processor and blend until smooth. Drink immediately.

Add a teaspoon of vanilla if you want a little more flavor without adding sugar.

Nutrition Facts (per serving):
Calories: 154 Fat: 0 Carbs: 21 Fiber: 0 Protein: 16

JUNE 2: APRICOT AND PEACH

Serves 2

This frosty and creamy smoothie is rich in stone fruit flavors and packs a wallop of skin-healthy carotenoids.

Ingredients:

1 frozen banana
½ cup apricot nectar
½ cup frozen peach
2 tablespoons chia seed
1 teaspoon lemon juice

Directions:

Combine all ingredients in a high-power blender or food processor and blend until smooth.
Drink immediately.

Apricot juice can be used in place of the pulp-rich apricot nectar if apricot nectar is unavailable.

Nutrition Facts (per serving):
Calories: 170 Fat: 5 Carbs: 26 Fiber: 8 Protein: 4

JUNE 3: APRICOT PEAR

Serves 2

This apricot and pear combination is exotic with the heady scent of turmeric.

Ingredients:

1 frozen banana

½ pear

½ cup apricot nectar

½ cup ice

2 tablespoons chia seed

½ teaspoon turmeric powder

Directions:

Combine all ingredients in a high-power blender or food processor and blend until smooth. Drink immediately.

Nutrition Facts (per serving):
Calories: 180 Fat: 5 Carbs: 29 Fiber: 9 Protein: 4

JUNE 4: APRICOT CHERRY SWIRL

Serves 1

This smoothie has sweet cherry and tart apricot flavors with a little citrus and vanilla finish.

Ingredients:

½ cup apricot nectar

½ cup frozen cherries

1 tablespoon chia seed

1 teaspoon lemon juice

½ teaspoon vanilla extract

Directions:

Combine all ingredients in a high-power blender or food processor and blend until smooth.

Drink immediately.

Nutrition Facts (per serving):
Calories: 189 Fat: 5 Carbs: 29 Fiber: 8 Protein: 4

JUNE 5: SPICED APRICOT

Serves 1

This medicinal elixir is a powerful blend of spices that triggers weight loss. The black pepper works synergistically with turmeric to help stimulate the release of extra water weight.

Ingredients:

½ cup apricot nectar

½ cup ice

1 tablespoon chia seed

¼ teaspoon turmeric powder

1 pinch of cardamom

1 pinch of fresh ground black pepper

Directions:

Combine all ingredients in a high-power blender or food processor and blend until smooth.

Drink immediately.

CULINARY TIP

If you're not yet used to spicy smoothies, you might want to start with just a pinch of each spice until you're used to them.

Nutrition Facts (per serving):
Calories: 135 Fat: 5 Carbs: 17 Fiber: 6 Protein: 3

JUNE 6: APRICOT FROSTY

Serves 2

This frosty blend is tart and spicy with a sweet hint of date.

Ingredients:

1 Medjool date

½ cup apricot nectar

½ cup frozen blackberries

½ cup frozen peach

2 tablespoons chia seed

1 pinch of fresh ground black pepper

1 pinch of cardamom

Directions:

Combine all ingredients in a high-power blender or food processor and blend until smooth. Drink immediately.

Nutrition Facts (per serving):
Calories: 174 Fat: 5 Carbs: 27 Fiber: 9 Protein: 4

JUNE 7: APRICOT CINNAMON CREAM

Serves 2

This frosty fruit blend is slightly sweet with a hint of cinnamon.

Ingredients:

½ frozen banana

½ cup apricot nectar

½ cup frozen raspberries

½ cup ice

2 tablespoons chia seed

1 pinch of ground cinnamon

Directions:

Combine all ingredients in a high-power blender or food processor and blend until smooth. Drink immediately.

CULINARY TIP

Nectars, such as the apricot nectar used here, are ideal for smoothies as they have a richer flavor and more pulp than juices.

Nutrition Facts (per serving):
Calories: 144 Fat: 5 Carbs: 19 Fiber: 9 Protein: 4

AVOCADO SMOOTHIES

JUNE 8: COCOA ALMOND CRUSH

Serves 2

This super-creamy smoothie has a little charge of cocoa. The unsweetened dark cocoa contains flavonoids that help reduce weight gain by improving the way our bodies utilize insulin.

Ingredients:

½ frozen banana

1 cup almond milk

½ cup ice

½ cup avocado

2 tablespoons chia seed

1 teaspoon unsweetened dark cocoa powder

1 teaspoon vanilla extract

Directions:

Combine all ingredients in a high-power blender or food processor and blend until smooth. Drink immediately.

CULINARY

TIP *Avocado adds a rich creaminess to smoothies and helps emulsify the ingredients so they don't separate in the glass. Plus, avocados taste amazing!*

Nutrition Facts (per serving):
Calories: 189 Fat: 12 Carbs: 13 Fiber: 10 Protein: 5

JUNE 9: THE ISLANDER

Serves 2

This drink has papaya flavor in a creamy, fresh avocado base. Avocados contain monounsaturated fatty acids, which are healthy fats that improve fat burning, especially in the abdominal area.

Ingredients:

½ cup papaya nectar

½ cup ice

½ cup avocado

2 tablespoons chia seed

½ teaspoon lime juice

Directions:

Combine all ingredients in a high-power blender or food processor and blend until smooth. Drink immediately.

CULINARY TIP *Lime juice is the perfect flavor pairing with papaya.*

Nutrition Facts (per serving):
Calories: 171 Fat: 10 Carbs: 13 Fiber: 9 Protein: 4

JUNE 10: COCONUT AVOCADO LIME

Serves 2

This smoothie is rich and thick with a light lime flavor.

Ingredients:

½ frozen banana

½ cup coconut water

½ cup avocado

½ cup nonfat Greek yogurt

1 teaspoon lime juice

Directions:

Combine all ingredients in a high-power blender
or food processor and blend until smooth.
Drink immediately.

Nutrition Facts (per serving):
Calories: 139 Fat: 5 Carbs: 16 Fiber: 4 Protein: 8

JUNE 11: GREEN LUSHY

Serves 2

This blend is silky and sweet and so good for you!

Ingredients:

1 banana

½ cup coconut water

½ cup avocado

½ cup frozen sweet cherries

2 tablespoons chia seed

Directions:

Combine all ingredients in a high-power blender
or food processor and blend until smooth.
Drink immediately.

Nutrition Facts (per serving):
Calories: 226 Fat: 10 Carbs: 28 Fiber: 12 Protein: 5

JUNE 12: FAUX PEACH

Serves 2

Surprise your taste buds with this date-sweetened green drink that is rich in antioxidants.

Ingredients:

1 tomato

1 Medjool date

½ cup unfiltered apple juice

½ cup ice

¼ cup avocado

2 tablespoons chia seed

Directions:

Combine all ingredients in a high-power blender or food processor and blend until smooth.
Drink immediately.

Nutrition Facts (per serving):
Calories: 177 Fat: 8 Carbs: 22 Fiber: 9 Protein: 4

JUNE 13: TULSI AVOCADO CREAM

Serves 2

This is a savory herbal smoothie with just a touch of sweetness from the date.

Ingredients:

1 Medjool date

½ cup hemp milk

½ cup ice

½ cup cucumber

¼ cup avocado

¼ cup fresh holy basil (tulsi) leaves

2 tablespoons chia seed

Directions:

Combine all ingredients in a high-power blender or food processor and blend until smooth. Drink immediately.

Nutrition Facts (per serving):
Calories: 179 Fat: 9 Carbs: 18 Fiber: 9 Protein: 5

CHERRY SMOOTHIES

JUNE 14: HAZELNUT CHERRY

Serves 1

Cherry, hazelnut and vanilla mingle beautifully in this cool, frosty concoction.

Ingredients:

½ cup hazelnut milk

½ cup ice

½ cup cherries

2 tablespoons vanilla-flavored protein powder

Directions:

Combine all ingredients in a high-power blender or food processor and blend until smooth. Drink immediately.

CULINARY TIP *Frozen cherries are pre-pitted, so you won't have to take the extra step of pitting them as you would with fresh cherries.*

Nutrition Facts (per serving):
Calories: 148 Fat: 2 Carbs: 23 Fiber: 2 Protein: 10

JUNE 15: VANILLA CHERRY FREEZE

Serves 1

This frosty, sweet cherry freeze has rich fruity flavor and vanilla fragrance.

Ingredients:

1 ½ cups frozen cherries

½ cup coconut water

½ cup nonfat Greek yogurt

2 tablespoons vanilla-flavored protein powder

1 teaspoon vanilla extract

Directions:

Combine all ingredients in a high-power blender or food processor and blend until smooth. Drink immediately.

Nutrition Facts (per serving):
Calories: 186 Fat: 1 Carbs: 30 Fiber: 5 Protein: 15

JUNE 16: CHERRY CITRUS SPICE

Serves 1

This rich cherry blend has a little citrus and spice.

Ingredients:

½ cup black cherry juice

½ cup frozen cherries

1 tablespoon chia seed

½ teaspoon lemon juice

1 pinch of fresh ground black pepper

Directions:

Combine all ingredients in a high-power blender or food processor and blend until smooth. Drink immediately.

Nutrition Facts (per serving):
Calories: 183 Fat: 5 Carbs: 29 Fiber: 8 Protein: 5

JUNE 17: SOUR CHERRY VANILLA

Serves 1

This creamy and rich combination is only slightly sweet with a little sour-cherry edge. Cherries contain antioxidant anthocyanins that help reduce pain resulting from inflammation.

Ingredients:

½ cup hemp milk

½ cup ice

½ cup nonfat Greek yogurt

½ cup frozen sour cherries

2 tablespoons vanilla-flavored protein powder

Directions:

Combine all ingredients in a high-power blender or food processor and blend until smooth. Drink immediately.

CULINARY TIP *Sour, dark or sweet whole cherries or black cherry juice can be used interchangeably in this recipe, as all contain anthocyanins.*

Nutrition Facts (per serving):
Calories: 115 Fat: 2 Carbs: 14 Fiber: 1 Protein: 11

JUNE 18: GRAPE CHERRY DREAM

Serves 2

This dreamy drink is sweet and fruity with layers of flavor. Resveratrol, found in grapes, can help protect the skin from sun-induced damage that can lead to cancer.

Ingredients:

½ cup grape juice

½ cup seedless grapes

½ cup ice

½ cup frozen tart cherries

2 tablespoons protein powder

1 teaspoon lemon juice

Directions:

Combine all ingredients in a high-power blender or food processor and blend until smooth. Drink immediately.

CULINARY TIP *The sweetness of grape juice complements the tartness of fruits such as tart cherries and pomegranate.*

Nutrition Facts (per serving):
Calories: 110 Fat: 0 Carbs: 23 Fiber: 1 Protein: 5

JUNE 19: CHERRY PINEAPPLE

Serves 2

This smoothie is the perfect balance of pineapple and cherries with a little vanilla and enough protein to energize you for a few hours.

Ingredients:

½ cup coconut water

½ cup frozen cherries

½ cup pineapple

½ cup ice

2 tablespoons vanilla-flavored protein powder

Directions:

Combine all ingredients in a high-power blender
or food processor and blend until smooth.
Drink immediately.

Nutrition Facts (per serving):
Calories: 77 Fat: 0 Carbs: 15 Fiber: 1 Protein: 5

JUNE 20: SPICED CHERRY REFRESHER

Serves 1

Hot and heady spices complement the sweet cherries
and citrus in this refreshing blend.

Ingredients:

½ cup coconut water

½ cup frozen sweet cherries

1 tablespoon chia seed

1 teaspoon lemon juice

1 pinch of cardamom

1 pinch of fresh ground black pepper

Directions:

Combine all ingredients in a high-power blender
or food processor and blend until smooth.
Drink immediately.

Nutrition Facts (per serving):
Calories: 139 Fat: 5 Carbs: 19 Fiber: 8 Protein: 4

PEACH SMOOTHIES

JUNE 21: PEACH BERRY

Serves 2

This peachy drink is light and fresh with a little citrus note. The coconut water is an ideal smoothie base because it doesn't have added sugar or food colorings, and it's low in calories and rich in electrolytes.

Ingredients:

1 peach

½ cup coconut water

½ cup frozen wild blackberries

2 tablespoons protein powder

1 teaspoon lemon juice

Directions:

Combine all ingredients in a high-power blender or food processor and blend until smooth.
Drink immediately.

Nutrition Facts (per serving):
Calories: 87 Fat: 0 Carbs: 15 Fiber: 3 Protein: 5

JUNE 22: GINGERED PEACH

Serves 2

Enjoy the peach flavor that is not too sweet thanks to a little heat from the ginger.

Ingredients:

1 peach

½ frozen banana

½ cup coconut water

½ cup ice

2 tablespoons chia seed

1 teaspoon fresh ginger root

Directions:

Combine all ingredients in a high-power blender or food processor and blend until smooth. Drink immediately.

CULINARY TIP *Use filtered water when making ice so that your ice will be free of contaminants and toxins.*

Nutrition Facts (per serving):
Calories: 132 Fat: 5 Carbs: 17 Fiber: 8 Protein: 4

JUNE 23: PEACHY BANANA

Serves 2

This enticing combination is creamy with layers of flavor. Peaches contain ellagic acid, a potent antioxidant being studied for its health-promoting benefits.

Ingredients:

1 peach
½ frozen banana
½ cup coconut water
½ cup hemp milk
¼ cup frozen cherries
¼ cup ice
2 tablespoons chia seed

Directions:

Combine all ingredients in a high-power blender or food processor and blend until smooth. Drink immediately.

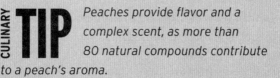

CULINARY TIP *Peaches provide flavor and a complex scent, as more than 80 natural compounds contribute to a peach's aroma.*

Nutrition Facts (per serving):
Calories: 178 Fat: 6 Carbs: 25 Fiber: 8 Protein: 5

JUNE 24: CHERRY VANILLA PEACH

Serves 2

This delicious combination is creamy and sweet and has layers of flavors. The yogurt provides protein, which reduces cravings, helps stabilize blood sugar and provides the amino acids needed for long-lasting energy.

Ingredients:

½ cup hazelnut milk
½ cup frozen cherries
½ cup frozen peaches
½ cup nonfat Greek yogurt
1 teaspoon vanilla extract

Directions:

Combine all ingredients in a high-power blender or food processor and blend until smooth. Drink immediately.

CULINARY TIP *Look for yogurt with less than 10 grams of sugar per serving.*

Nutrition Facts (per serving):
Calories: 106 Fat: 1 Carbs: 17 Fiber: 2 Protein: 7

DONUT PEACH SMOOTHIES

JUNE 25: GINGERED DONUT PEACH

Serves 2

Try this delightful combination of sweet peaches with a little heat and citrus. The ginger root has a warming effect, which stimulates and supports digestion.

Ingredients:

2 donut peaches

½ cup coconut water

½ cup ice

2 tablespoons chia seed

1 tablespoon fresh ginger root

1 teaspoon lemon juice

Directions:

Combine all ingredients in a high-power blender or food processor and blend until smooth.

Drink immediately.

CULINARY TIP *Fresh ginger root is available in most grocery stores. Break off a 1-inch chunk of root, cut off the outer skin and chop before adding to the blender.*

Nutrition Facts (per serving):
Calories: 133 Fat: 5 Carbs: 7 Fiber: 8 Protein: 4

JUNE 26: CINNAMON PEACH

Serves 2

You'll love the donut peaches' lusciousness with a little vanilla and cinnamon. One study found that participants who took a ½ teaspoon of cinnamon per day were able to control cholesterol and triglyceride levels without medication.

Ingredients:

2 donut peaches
½ cup coconut water
½ cup ice
½ cup nonfat Greek yogurt
1 tablespoon vanilla-flavored protein powder
¼ teaspoon ground cinnamon

Directions:

Combine all ingredients in a high-power blender or food processor and blend until smooth. Drink immediately.

CULINARY TIP *Add a teaspoon of xylitol to sweeten if desired.*

Nutrition Facts (per serving):
Calories: 105 Fat: 0 Carbs: 18 Fiber: 2 Protein: 9

JUNE 27: CILANTRO PEACH ORANGE

Serves 2

This smoothie has fresh cilantro fragrance in a sweet orange juice and fresh peach base.

Ingredients:

2 donut peaches

½ cup orange juice

½ cup ice

¼ cup cilantro leaves

2 tablespoon hulled hemp seed

Directions:

Combine all ingredients in a high-power blender
or food processor and blend until smooth.
Drink immediately.

Nutrition Facts (per serving):
Calories: 123 Fat: 3 Carbs: 20 Fiber: 3 Protein: 4

JUNE 28: SPICED ORANGE PEACH

Serves 2

This smoothie has a citrus base with a little spice.

Ingredients:

2 donut peaches

½ navel orange

1 cup orange juice

½ cup ice

2 tablespoons whey protein

1 pinch of ground clove

Directions:

Combine all ingredients in a high-power blender
or food processor and blend until smooth.
Drink immediately.

Nutrition Facts (per serving):
Calories: 145 Fat: 1 Carbs: 30 Fiber: 3 Protein: 7

JUNE 29: BASIL ORANGE PEACH

Serves 2

Try this herbed orange smoothie with a little lime and a lot of fat-burning power.

Ingredients:

2 donut peaches

½ cup coconut water

½ cup orange juice

½ cup ice

¼ cup fresh holy basil leaves

2 tablespoons hulled hemp seed

1 teaspoon lime juice

½ teaspoon turmeric powder

Directions:

Combine all ingredients in a high-power blender or food processor and blend until smooth. Drink immediately.

Nutrition Facts (per serving):
Calories: 134 Fat: 3 Carbs: 23 Fiber: 3 Protein: 4

JUNE 30: SPICED HIBISCUS BERRY

Serves 2

This smoothie provides a refreshing blend of bright red tea and berry flavors. The black pepper and cardamom help stimulate healthy immune function and taste amazing in smoothies!

Ingredients:

2 donut peaches

1 cup brewed hibiscus tea

1 cup frozen wild blueberries

½ cup ice

¼ cup pomegranate juice

2 tablespoons chia seed

1 pinch of ground cardamom

1 pinch of fresh ground black pepper

....

Directions:

Combine all ingredients in a high-power blender
or food processor and blend until smooth.
Drink immediately.

....

Nutrition Facts (per serving):
Calories: 154 Fat: 5 Carbs: 22 Fiber: 10 Protein: 4

CHAPTER 10

July Smoothies

BLACK CHERRY JUICE SMOOTHIES

JULY 1: CHOCOLATE CHERRY

Serves 2

This sweet cherry blend includes coconut and rich vanilla flavor throughout.

Ingredients:

½ frozen banana

½ cup coconut water

½ cup frozen tart cherries

¼ cup black cherry juice

2 tablespoons vanilla-flavored protein powder

1 tablespoon unsweetened cocoa powder

Directions:

Combine all ingredients in a high-power blender or food processor and blend until smooth.

Drink immediately.

Nutrition Facts (per serving):
Calories: 92 Fat: 0 Carbs: 18 Fiber: 1 Protein: 5

JULY 2: BERRY MANGO TART

Serves 2

This creamy blueberry-rich drink offers a tart citrus flavor to the palate.

Ingredients:

1 cup frozen blueberries

½ cup frozen mango

½ cup nonfat Greek yogurt

¼ cup black cherry juice

1 teaspoon lemon juice

Directions:

Combine all ingredients in a high-power blender or food processor and blend until smooth. Drink immediately.

Nutrition Facts (per serving):
Calories: 110 Fat: 0 Carbs: 22 Fiber: 4 Protein: 7

JULY 3: DOUBLE CHERRY

Serves 1

This recipe calls for black cherry juice, which is rich in anti-inflammatory anthocyanins. Much of what we think of as body fat is actually inflammation that can be reduced by natural anti-inflammatories from foods such as cherries. With the higher calorie count, this smoothie can be considered a meal-replacement smoothie instead of a snack.

Ingredients:

½ frozen banana

½ cup black cherry juice

½ cup frozen cherries

2 tablespoons hulled hemp seed

Directions:

Combine all ingredients in a high-power blender or food processor and blend until smooth. Drink immediately.

Nutrition Facts (per serving):
Calories: 255 Fat: 6 Carbs: 44 Fiber: 5 Protein: 7

CHERRY TOMATO SMOOTHIES

JULY 4: APPLE TOMATO DATE

Serves 2

This drink tastes like a tomato-yogurt bisque and is sweetened with a date.

Ingredients:

1 Medjool date

½ cup unfiltered apple juice

½ cup ice

½ cup cherry tomatoes

½ cup nonfat Greek yogurt

Directions:

Combine all ingredients in a high-power blender or food processor and blend until smooth. Drink immediately.

Nutrition Facts (per serving):
Calories: 101 Fat: 0 Carbs: 20 Fiber: 1 Protein: 7

JULY 5: TOMATO KICKER

Serves 2

This tomato smoothie is fresh and cool with a touch of heat in the back of the throat. Carotenoid antioxidants in hot peppers protect healthy cells from oxidative stress, and a daily dose can help protect us from wrinkles, cancer and other oxidative imbalances.

Ingredients:

½ cucumber
½ cup cherry tomatoes
½ cup ice
¼ cup medium-hot pepper
2 tablespoons chia seed

Directions:

Combine all ingredients in a high-power blender or food processor and blend until smooth. Drink immediately.

CULINARY TIP *Choose peppers with the level of heat that you prefer.*

Nutrition Facts (per serving):
Calories: 90 Fat: 5 Carbs: 5 Fiber: 7 Protein: 4

JULY 6: FRESH BLOODY MARY

Serves 1

Have one of these to kick-start your morning!

Ingredients:

1 celery stalk

1 cup cherry tomatoes

½ cup ice

1 tablespoon lemon juice

½ teaspoon horseradish

½ teaspoon Tabasco

1 pinch of fresh ground black pepper

1 pinch of celery salt

1 pinch of cayenne

Directions:

Combine all ingredients in a high-power blender
or food processor and blend until smooth.
Drink immediately.

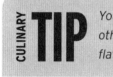

CULINARY TIP *You can also add any of your other favorite Bloody Mary flavors to this recipe.*

Nutrition Facts (per serving):
Calories: 29 Fat: 0 Carbs: 7 Fiber: 2 Protein: 1

JULY 7: SUMMERTIME SLIMMER

Serves 2

Enjoy fresh-from-the-garden summertime flavor
in this smoothie.

Ingredients:

½ cup carrot juice

½ cup ice

½ cup basil leaves

½ cup cherry tomatoes

2 tablespoons chia seed

Directions:

Combine all ingredients in a high-power blender
or food processor and blend until smooth.
Drink immediately.

Nutrition Facts (per serving):
Calories: 101 Fat: 5 Carbs: 8 Fiber: 7 Protein: 4

FRESH FIG SMOOTHIES

JULY 8: APPLE CHERRY FIG

Serves 2

This drink is intensely sweet with warm vanilla
and fig undertones.

Ingredients:

1 fig

½ cup unfiltered apple juice

½ cup nonfat Greek yogurt

½ cup frozen cherries

½ vanilla bean

½ teaspoon turmeric powder

Directions:

Combine all ingredients in a high-power blender
or food processor and blend until smooth.
Drink immediately.

Nutrition Facts (per serving):
Calories: 104 Fat: 0 Carbs: 20 Fiber: 2 Protein: 7

JULY 9: HAZELNUT FIG WHIP

Serves 1

This smoothie combines a creamy banana flavor with a little fig.

Ingredients:

1 fig

½ frozen banana

½ cup hazelnut milk

½ cup ice

2 tablespoons hulled hemp seed

Directions:

Combine all ingredients in a high-power blender or food processor and blend until smooth.
Drink immediately.

Nutrition Facts (per serving):
Calories: 234 Fat: 8 Carbs: 36 Fiber: 5 Protein: 7

JULY 10: SPICED ALMOND CREAM

Serves 1

This creamy vanilla-based smoothie is gratifying, with a hint of fig and spices.

Ingredients:

1 fig

½ cup almond milk

½ cup ice

½ cup nonfat Greek yogurt

½ teaspoon vanilla extract

1 pinch of cinnamon

1 pinch of fresh ground black pepper

Directions:
Combine all ingredients in a high-power blender
or food processor and blend until smooth.
Drink immediately.

Nutrition Facts (per serving):
Calories: 125 Fat: 1 Carbs: 15 Fiber: 1 Protein: 13

HONEYDEW MELON SMOOTHIES

JULY 11: SWEET TEA

Serves 2

Lightly brewed green tea provides a nutrient-rich
base for this melon smoothie. Green tea contains
antioxidant compounds that are being studied for
their potential as weight loss nutrients.

Ingredients:
½ frozen banana
1 cup brewed green tea
½ cup honeydew melon
2 tablespoons chia seed

Directions:
Combine all ingredients in a high-power blender
or food processor and blend until smooth.
Drink immediately.

CULINARY TIP *Brew green tea regularly and keep it on hand for smoothie making or freeze it in ice cube trays to add to smoothies.*

Nutrition Facts (per serving):
Calories: 111 Fat: 5 Carbs: 12 Fiber: 7 Protein: 4

JULY 12: MELON CITRUS

Serves 2

This citrus smoothie combines a sweet watermelon flavor with tangy lime.

Ingredients:

1 cup watermelon

½ cup honeydew melon

½ cup ice

2 tablespoons chia seed

1 teaspoon lime juice

½ teaspoon turmeric powder

Directions:

Combine all ingredients in a high-power blender or food processor and blend until smooth.
Drink immediately.

Nutrition Facts (per serving):
Calories: 107 Fat: 5 Carbs: 11 Fiber: 7 Protein: 4

JULY 13: MELON TEA FREEZE

Serves 2

This is a light, revitalizing smoothie and a healthy alternative to a margarita!

Ingredients:

2 cups honeydew melon

1 cup brewed green tea

½ cup ice

2 tablespoons hulled hemp seed

Directions:

Combine all ingredients in a high-power blender or food processor and blend until smooth.
Drink immediately.

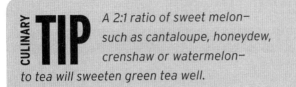

A 2:1 ratio of sweet melon—
such as cantaloupe, honeydew,
crenshaw or watermelon—
to tea will sweeten green tea well.

Nutrition Facts (per serving):
Calories: 106 Fat: 3 Carbs: 17 Fiber: 2 Protein: 3

JULY 14: SVELTE SYNERGY

Serves 2

This frosty coconut and melon power blend will kick-start your energy. The minerals in the coconut water and the protein in the hemp seed may be just what you need when your energy starts to lag during the day.

Ingredients:

1 cup honeydew melon

1 cup coconut water

½ cup brewed green tea

½ cup ice

2 tablespoons hulled hemp seed

Directions:

Combine all ingredients in a high-power blender or food processor and blend until smooth. Drink immediately.

Use a ½ teaspoon of orange or vanilla extract to punch up the flavor.

Nutrition Facts (per serving):
Calories: 97 Fat: 3 Carbs: 15 Fiber: 2 Protein: 3

FRESH KIWI SMOOTHIES

JULY 15: KIWI QUENCHER

Serves 2

This fresh kiwi smoothie combines sweet melon with intense kiwi flavor and a bit of citrus.

Ingredients:

1 kiwi

1 cup cantaloupe

½ cup water

½ cup ice

2 tablespoons chia seed

½ teaspoon lemon juice

Directions:

Combine all ingredients in a high-power blender or food processor and blend until smooth. Drink immediately.

Nutrition Facts (per serving):
Calories: 118 Fat: 5 Carbs: 13 Fiber: 8 Protein: 4

JULY 16: KIWI STRAWBERRY AND CHIA

Serves 2

This berry and kiwi blend is the perfect balance of sweet and tart.

Ingredients:

1 kiwi

1 cup frozen strawberries

½ cup coconut water

½ cup ice

2 tablespoons chia seed

Directions:

Combine all ingredients in a high-power blender or food processor and blend until smooth. Drink immediately.

CULINARY TIP *If you like a tart flavor, use two kiwis in this recipe.*

Nutrition Facts (per serving):
Calories: 127 Fat: 5 Carbs: 16 Fiber: 9 Protein: 4

JULY 17: KIWI APPLE

Serves 1

This refreshing treat is tart and sweet with citrus undertones.

Ingredients:

1 kiwi

½ cup unfiltered apple juice

½ cup ice

2 tablespoons protein powder

1 teaspoon lemon juice

¼ teaspoon turmeric powder

Directions:

Combine all ingredients in a high-power blender or food processor and blend until smooth. Drink immediately.

Nutrition Facts (per serving):
Calories: 144 Fat: 1 Carbs: 25 Fiber: 2 Protein: 9

JULY 18: KIWI BANANA

Serves 2

In this drink, you'll find an intense blend of tart and creamy with chia protein.

Ingredients:

1 kiwi

1 frozen banana

½ cup coconut water

½ cup ice

2 tablespoons chia seed

Directions:

Combine all ingredients in a high-power blender or food processor and blend until smooth. Drink immediately.

Nutrition Facts (per serving):

Calories: 154 Fat: 5 Carbs: 22 Fiber: 9 Protein: 4

FRESH TOMATO SMOOTHIES

JULY 19: SKINNY GINGER

Serves 2

This veggie-based drink comes alive with the flavors of mint and ginger. The cucumbers contain phytonutrients called cucurbitacins, which are being studied for their immune-supporting benefits.

Ingredients:

1 tomato

½ cucumber

½ cup coconut water

½ cup ice

2 tablespoons chia seed

1 tablespoon fresh mint leaves

1 tablespoon fresh ginger root

Directions:
Combine all ingredients in a high-power blender
or food processor and blend until smooth.
Drink immediately.

CULINARY TIP *Fresh mint leaves have a strong scent
and impart intense flavor to recipes,
but dried mint leaves can be used
instead, as they are widely available and have a
longer shelf life.*

Nutrition Facts (per serving):
Calories: 99 Fat: 5 Carbs: 8 Fiber: 7 Protein: 4

JULY 20: PARADISE IN A GLASS

Serves 2

The ingredients here create a creamy drink with fresh
avocado flavor.

Ingredients:
1 tomato

1 cup unfiltered apple juice

½ cup ice

½ cup avocado

2 tablespoons chia seed

1 tablespoon lemon juice

Directions:
Combine all ingredients in a high-power blender
or food processor and blend until smooth.
Drink immediately.

Nutrition Facts (per serving):
Calories: 207 Fat: 10 Carbs: 22 Fiber: 10 Protein: 5

JULY 21: MINTY V-3

Serves 1

This is a simple veggie smoothie perfect for those easing their way into green smoothies. Additionally, tomato juice can help the body clear excess (unhealthy) LDL cholesterol.

Ingredients:

½ cup carrot juice

½ cup ice

¼ cup tomato

¼ cup fresh mint leaves

1 tablespoon chia seed

Directions:

Combine all ingredients in a high-power blender or food processor and blend until smooth. Drink immediately.

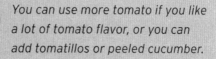

CULINARY TIP *You can use more tomato if you like a lot of tomato flavor, or you can add tomatillos or peeled cucumber.*

Nutrition Facts (per serving):
Calories: 129 Fat: 5 Carbs: 15 Fiber: 8 Protein: 5

JULY 22: LOVE APPLE

Serves 2

This drink has a fresh and healthy flavor, and the holy basil found here is used medicinally in India to prevent blood sugar imbalance.

Ingredients:

½ cup ice

½ cup unfiltered apple juice

½ cup tomato

¼ cup fresh holy basil leaves

2 tablespoons chia seed

½ teaspoon lemon juice

Directions:

Combine all ingredients in a high-power blender or food processor and blend until smooth. Drink immediately.

CULINARY TIP *Fresh holy basil is preferable, but dried is more widely available and requires a smaller portion (just 1 teaspoon).*

Nutrition Facts (per serving):
Calories: 107 Fat: 5 Carbs: 10 Fiber: 7 Protein: 4

FRESH APRICOT SMOOTHIES

JULY 23: TART BANANA

Serves 2

This smoothie's fresh fruit flavor combines well with the creaminess of the frozen banana, and the apricots have a slight tartness that complements the sweetness of the rich blueberry nectar.

Ingredients:

2 apricots

½ frozen banana

½ cup blueberry nectar

2 tablespoons chia seed

Directions:

Combine all ingredients in a high-power blender or food processor and blend until smooth. Drink immediately.

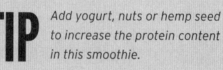

CULINARY TIP *Add yogurt, nuts or hemp seed to increase the protein content in this smoothie.*

Nutrition Facts (per serving):
Calories: 145 Fat: 5 Carbs: 19 Fiber: 7 Protein: 4

JULY 24: BLACK VELVET APRICOT

Serves 2

Here you'll taste a tart and complex drink with rich apricot flavor.

Ingredients:

2 black velvet apricots

½ cup coconut water

½ cup ice

½ cup blueberry nectar

2 tablespoons chia seed

Directions:

Combine all ingredients in a high-power blender or food processor and blend until smooth. Drink immediately.

CULINARY TIP *You can replace the black velvet apricots with other types of apricots or other types of stone-fruits to make variations of this smoothie.*

Nutrition Facts (per serving):
Calories: 129 Fat: 5 Carbs: 15 Fiber: 7 Protein: 3

JULY 25: APRICOT APPLE

Serves 2

Apple, apricot and banana flavors create a not-too-sweet, rich and frosty blend.

Ingredients:

1 apricot

1 frozen banana

½ cup unfiltered apple juice

½ cup ice

2 tablespoons chia seed

Directions:

Combine all ingredients in a high-power blender or food processor and blend until smooth. Drink immediately.

CULINARY TIP *Adding ice to smoothies provides a frosty texture and more water for hydration, but it also dilutes the flavors a bit and is not necessary. Smoothie enthusiasts seem to either love or hate the addition of ice. You decide.*

Nutrition Facts (per serving):
Calories: 159 Fat: 5 Carbs: 23 Fiber: 8 Protein: 4

JULY 26: FRESH APRICOT

Serves 1

The light fruit flavor of this combination has a nutty bite with a twist of citrus.

Ingredients:

½ cup water

½ cup apricot

½ cup ice

2 tablespoons cashews

1 teaspoon lemon juice

Directions:

Combine all ingredients in a high-power blender or food processor and blend until smooth. Drink immediately.

CULINARY TIP Use any fruit with nuts and lemon, and you are bound to come up with a nice combination. The cashews in this smoothie are a good source of protein, but they also contain fat. Therefore, when adding nuts to smoothies, aim for 2 tablespoons per serving of smoothie for maximum nutrition.

Nutrition Facts (per serving):
Calories: 165 Fat: 11 Carbs: 11 Fiber: 1 Protein: 5

JULY 27: TULSI ORANGE

Serves 2

You'll taste orange infused with herbs in this cool and creamy blend.

Ingredients:

½ cup orange juice

½ cup apricot

½ cup ice

½ cup nonfat Greek yogurt

¼ cup fresh holy basil (tulsi) leaves

2 tablespoons hulled hemp seed

Directions:

Combine all ingredients in a high-power blender or food processor and blend until smooth. Drink immediately.

Nutrition Facts (per serving):
Calories: 125 Fat: 3 Carbs: 15 Fiber: 2 Protein: 10

WATERMELON SMOOTHIES

JULY 28: WATERMELON LEMONADE

Serves 2

Watermelon takes the center stage in this refreshing blend.

Ingredients:

½ frozen banana

1 cup ice

1 cup watermelon

½ cup coconut water

2 tablespoons chia seed

1 tablespoon lemon juice

Directions:

Combine all ingredients in a high-power blender or food processor and blend until smooth. Drink immediately.

Nutrition Facts (per serving):
Calories: 129 Fat: 5 Carbs: 16 Fiber: 7 Protein: 4

JULY 29: MINT MELON MOJITO

Serves 1

Watermelon and mint are the perfect pairing and give this smoothie its luxurious flavor, while lycopene and antioxidants in the watermelon help protect the skin from cancer.

Ingredients:

½ cup coconut water

½ cup watermelon

½ cup ice

¼ cup fresh mint leaves

2 tablespoons chia seed

1 tablespoon lime juice

Directions:

Combine all ingredients in a high-power blender
or food processor and blend until smooth.

Drink immediately.

CULINARY TIP

Fresh watermelon is key to the flavor of this smoothie.

Nutrition Facts (per serving):
Calories: 187 Fat: 10 Carbs: 14 Fiber: 13 Protein: 7

JULY 30: MINT WATERMELON

Serves 2

This blend is surprisingly sweet, tasty and refreshing,
with a strong watermelon flavor.

Ingredients:

5 fresh holy basil leaves

1 cup watermelon

½ cup ice

½ cup unfiltered apple juice

¼ cup fresh mint leaves

2 tablespoons chia seed

Directions:

Combine all ingredients in a high-power blender
or food processor and blend until smooth.

Drink immediately.

Nutrition Facts (per serving):
Calories: 123 Fat: 5 Carbs: 14 Fiber: 7 Protein: 4

JULY 31: COCONUT WATERMELON BANANA

Serves 2

This refreshing treat offers an indulgent and healthy taste of the tropics.

Ingredients:

½ cup coconut water

½ cup watermelon

½ cup frozen banana

½ cup ice

½ cup nonfat Greek yogurt

1 tablespoon unsweetened fine macaroon coconut

Directions:

Combine all ingredients in a high-power blender or food processor and blend until smooth.

Drink immediately.

Nutrition Facts (per serving):
Calories: 97 Fat: 2 Carbs: 15 Fiber: 1 Protein: 7

CHAPTER 11

August Smoothies

WILD BLUEBERRY SMOOTHIES

AUGUST 1: BLUEBERRY CHERRY TART

Serves 1

This drink combines tart, bright fruit flavors in a frosty blend.

Ingredients:

½ cup blueberry nectar

½ cup ice

½ cup frozen cherries

¼ cup wild blueberries

Directions:

Combine all ingredients in a high-power blender or food processor and blend until smooth. Drink immediately.

CULINARY TIP *Add a little pineapple or apple juice if this combination is too tart for your taste. Wild blueberries have exceptionally high antioxidant levels and are sold in the freezer section of most grocery stores.*

Nutrition Facts (per serving):
Calories: 130 Fat: 0 Carbs: 33 Fiber: 3 Protein: 1

AUGUST 2: BLUEBERRY FAIRY

Serves 1

This tart, slightly sweet and refreshing smoothie is dense in antioxidant polyphenols, which give this drink its rich purple color.

Ingredients:

½ cup frozen wild blueberries

½ cup ice

½ cup blueberry nectar

1 tablespoon chia seed

Directions:

Combine all ingredients in a high-power blender or food processor and blend until smooth. Drink immediately.

Nutrition Facts (per serving):
Calories: 177 Fat: 5 Carbs: 27 Fiber: 6 Protein: 3

AUGUST 3: WILD BLUEBERRY QUENCHER

Serves 1

This smoothie is filled with tart, fresh, clear blueberry flavor.

Ingredients:

½ cup coconut water

½ cup frozen wild blueberries

½ cup ice

1 tablespoon hulled hemp seed

Directions:

Combine all ingredients in a high-power blender or food processor and blend until smooth. Drink immediately.

CULINARY TIP *Wild frozen blueberries are available in grocery stores year round, or you can pick them yourself if you have access to this intense little fruit.*

Nutrition Facts (per serving):

Calories: 108 Fat: 3 Carbs: 17 Fiber: 1 Protein: 3

AUGUST 4: KUL KAH HAN'S GARDEN

Serves 2

The pairing of fresh wild blueberries with vanilla is perfection in this recipe! It was inspired by the northwest native blueberries and huckleberries growing at Kul Kah Han's Native Plant Garden in Chimacum, Washington.

Ingredients:

½ cup coconut water

½ cup frozen wild blueberries

½ cup nonfat Greek yogurt

½ cup ice

2 tablespoons vanilla-flavored protein powder

Directions:

Combine all ingredients in a high-power blender or food processor and blend until smooth. Drink immediately.

CULINARY TIP *Wild berries—such as lingonberries, huckleberries, blackberries and blueberries—provide intense flavor for smoothies. All are available online via nwwildfoods.com.*

Nutrition Facts (per serving):
Calories: 84 Fat: 0 Carbs: 11 Fiber: 2 Protein: 10

AUGUST 5: WILD BLUEBERRY LIME

Serves 1

Wild berries have about twice the nutrient levels as cultivated berries and give this smoothie an intense blueberry flavor with just a bit of lime. Because of the higher calorie count, consider this a meal-replacement smoothie instead of a snack.

Ingredients:

½ cup coconut water

½ cup frozen wild blueberries

½ cup blueberry nectar

2 tablespoons chia seed

1 teaspoon lime juice

Directions:
Combine all ingredients in a high-power blender
or food processor and blend until smooth.
Drink immediately.

Nutrition Facts (per serving):
Calories: 261 Fat: 10 Carbs: 33 Fiber: 15 Protein: 6

MANGO NECTAR SMOOTHIES

AUGUST 6: BASIL MANGO

Serves 1

This recipe is a gentle blend of mango and basil.

Ingredients:
½ cup mango nectar
½ cup ice
½ cup frozen mango
¼ cup fresh holy basil leaves
2 tablespoons hulled hemp seed

Directions:
Combine all ingredients in a high-power blender
or food processor and blend until smooth.
Drink immediately.

Nutrition Facts (per serving):
Calories: 205 Fat: 6 Carbs: 31 Fiber: 3 Protein: 6

AUGUST 7: A TROPICAL ORANGE

Serves 1

This frosty blend is slightly tropical, with a little orange and vanilla flavor.

Ingredients:

1 navel orange

½ cup mango nectar

½ cup ice

2 tablespoons protein powder

½ teaspoon vanilla extract

Directions:

Combine all ingredients in a high-power blender or food processor and blend until smooth.
Drink immediately.

Nutrition Facts (per serving):
Calories: 184 Fat: 1 Carbs: 34 Fiber: 3 Protein: 10

AUGUST 8: AFTERNOON OASIS

Serves 2

This drink has bright flavors that each get their moment on the palate. Hulled hemp seed provides the smoothie with 5 grams of protein in just 2 tablespoons.

Ingredients:

1 cup mango nectar

½ cup ice

¼ cup frozen raspberries

¼ cup frozen cherries

2 tablespoons hulled hemp seed

Directions:

Combine all ingredients in a high-power blender
or food processor and blend until smooth.
Drink immediately.

Nutrition Facts (per serving):
Calories: 129 Fat: 3 Carbs: 22 Fiber: 2 Protein: 3

FRESH PAPAYA SMOOTHIES

AUGUST 9: PAPAYA CITRUS SOOTHER

Serves 1

This smoothie is light, fresh and easy to digest.
Papaya is an excellent source of carotenoids, which
are necessary for healthy skin.

Ingredients:

1 cup papaya

¼ cup water

¼ cup ice

1 tablespoon chia seed

1 teaspoon lemon juice

Directions:

Combine all ingredients in a high-power blender
or food processor and blend until smooth.
Drink immediately.

CULINARY TIP Remove the seeds and skin
of the papaya before adding
it to the smoothie.

Nutrition Facts (per serving):
Calories 132 Fat: 5 Carbs: 17 Fiber: 8 Protein: 4

AUGUST 10: PAPAYA LIME CRUSH

Serves 1

Papaya and lime are a heavenly combination.

Ingredients:

1 cup papaya

¼ cup water

¼ cup ice

1 tablespoon hulled hemp seed

1 teaspoon lime juice

Directions:

Combine all ingredients in a high-power blender or food processor and blend until smooth. Drink immediately.

CULINARY TIP *Frozen papaya is just as healthy as fresh, and it tastes great! If you'd like to boost the protein in this smoothie, simply toss in an additional tablespoon of hulled hemp seed.*

Nutrition Facts (per serving):
Calories: 107 Fat: 3 Carbs: 17 Fiber: 3 Protein: 3

AUGUST 11: PAPAYA LIME FIZZ

Serves 1

This perfect blend of papaya and lime is hydrating and a nice little afternoon energizer.

Ingredients:

1 cup papaya

2 tablespoons chia seed

1 tablespoon lime juice

1 cup sparkling water

Directions:

Combine papaya, chia seed and lime juice in a high-power blender or food processor and blend until smooth. Then, stir in the sparkling water and drink immediately.

CULINARY TIP *Filtered (flat) tap water can also be used instead of sparkling water and can be blended together with the other ingredients at the same time. If you do use sparkling water, be sure to add it **after** blending the rest of the ingredients, as blending bubbly water pops all the bubbles.*

Nutrition Facts (per serving):
Calories: 202 Fat: 10 Carbs: 18 Fiber: 14 Protein: 7

AUGUST 12: MAUI MORNING

Serves 2

This smoothie has an intense papaya and lime flavor.

Ingredients:

½ frozen banana

1 cup papaya

½ cup coconut water

½ cup ice

2 tablespoons chia seed

1 teaspoon lime juice

½ teaspoon turmeric powder

Directions:

Combine all ingredients in a high-power blender or food processor and blend until smooth.

Drink immediately.

Nutrition Facts (per serving):
Calories: 137 Fat: 5 Carbs: 18 Fiber: 8 Protein: 4

AUGUST 13: HAWAIIAN DREAM

Serves 2

This refreshing drink tastes like a sunny day on a Hawaiian beach.

Ingredients:

1 cup papaya

½ cup frozen pineapple

½ cup coconut water

½ cup ice

2 tablespoons protein powder

Directions:
Combine all ingredients in a high-power blender
or food processor and blend until smooth.
Drink immediately.

Nutrition Facts (per serving):
Calories 84 Fat: 0 Carbs: 17 Fiber: 2 Protein: 5

AUGUST 14: VANILLA MANDARIN

Serves 2

This blend has sweet Mandarin citrus and rich, exotic
papaya flavors with sweet blueberry high notes.

Ingredients:
1 Mandarin orange
½ cup papaya
½ cup frozen wild blueberries
½ cup ice
2 tablespoons chia seed
1 tablespoon lemon juice
½ teaspoon vanilla extract

Directions:
Combine all ingredients in a high-power blender
or food processor and blend until smooth.
Drink immediately.

Nutrition Facts (per serving):
Calories 126 Fat: 5 Carbs: 15 Fiber: 9 Protein: 3

AUGUST 15: PAPAYA MANGO LIME

Serves 2

The tropical flavors are complemented by the fresh lime in this smoothie. It tastes great, and the protein and essential fatty acids in hemp satisfy hunger.

Ingredients:

½ cup coconut water

½ cup papaya

½ cup mango

½ cup ice

2 tablespoons hulled hemp seed

1 teaspoon lime juice

Directions:

Combine all ingredients in a high-power blender or food processor and blend until smooth. Drink immediately.

CULINARY TIP *If you prefer smoother textures, you might opt for hemp protein powder in its softer protein powder form rather than hulled hemp seed, which are whole seeds.*

Nutrition Facts (per serving):
Calories: 95 Fat: 3 Carbs: 14 Fiber: 2 Protein: 3

AUGUST 16: CHERRY BLUE PAPAYA

Serves 2

Enjoy this sweet cherry base with just a little papaya and vanilla flavor.

Ingredients:

1 cup frozen sweet cherries

½ cup coconut water

½ cup blueberry nectar

½ cup papaya

2 tablespoons protein powder

½ teaspoon turmeric powder

½ teaspoon vanilla extract

Directions:

Combine all ingredients in a high-power blender or food processor and blend until smooth. Drink immediately.

Nutrition Facts (per serving):
Calories: 132 Fat: 0 Carbs: 27 Fiber: 2 Protein: 5

AUGUST 17: HOT PEPPER PAPAYA

Serves 2

This pink beauty has a fragrant pepper scent and a sweet strawberry flavor, as well as slight heat. Strawberries provide more vitamin C than citrus fruits and are rich in soluble fiber.

Ingredients:

1 cup frozen strawberries

½ cup brewed green tea

½ cup water

¼ cup papaya

¼ cup medium-hot pepper

2 tablespoons chia seed

Directions:

Combine all ingredients in a high-power blender or food processor and blend until smooth. Drink immediately.

CULINARY TIP *Strawberries with a deep red coloring are riper and sweeter and contain more nutrients than the less ripe berries with lighter coloring.*

Nutrition Facts (per serving):
Calories: 111 Fat: 5 Carbs: 11 Fiber: 8 Protein: 4

AUGUST 18: ORANGE PAPAYA LIME

Serves 2

This smoothie has a light, tropical citrus flavor.

Ingredients:

1 cup papaya

½ cup ice

½ cup orange juice

2 tablespoons chia seed

1 teaspoon lime juice

Directions:

Combine all ingredients in a high-power blender or food processor and blend until smooth.

Drink immediately.

Nutrition Facts (per serving):
Calories: 120 Fat: 5 Carbs: 15 Fiber: 7 Protein: 4

FRESH WATERMELON SMOOTHIES

AUGUST 19: WATERMELON BLUEBERRY

Serves 1

This delicious smoothie tastes like a sweet blueberry dessert. Exquisite!

Ingredients:

1 cup watermelon

½ cup blueberry nectar

1 tablespoon vanilla-flavored protein powder

Directions:

Combine all ingredients in a high-power blender or food processor and blend until smooth. Drink immediately.

Nutrition Facts (per serving):
Calories: 132 Fat: 0 Carbs: 28 Fiber: 1 Protein: 5

AUGUST 20: GINGER BERRY MELON

Serves 2

This blend is a simple yet perfect combination of sweet and spicy. Additionally, ginger may elevate mood, as it stimulates neurotransmitters in the gastrointestinal tract that make us feel happy.

Ingredients:

2 cups watermelon

1 cup frozen wild blueberries

½ cup ice

2 tablespoons chia seed

1 tablespoon fresh ginger root

Directions:

Combine all ingredients in a high-power blender or food processor and blend until smooth. Drink immediately.

CULINARY TIP *Fresh ginger root can be chopped or pressed through a garlic press to extract its flavorful juice.*

Nutrition Facts (per serving):
Calories: 153 Fat: 5 Carbs: 23 Fiber: 10 Protein: 4

AUGUST 21: WATERMELON BANANA CREAM

Serves 2

This blended drink is sweet and rich in fruit flavor.

Ingredients:

½ frozen banana

1 cup watermelon

½ cup papaya nectar

2 tablespoons chia seed

Directions:

Combine all ingredients in a high-power blender or food processor and blend until smooth. Drink immediately.

Nutrition Facts (per serving):
Calories: 151 Fat: 5 Carbs: 21 Fiber: 7 Protein: 4

AUGUST 22: HOT WATERMELON

Serves 2

Hot peppers are rich in vitamin C and carotene and make this a sweet and fresh drink with a little heat on the palate.

Ingredients:

1 cup watermelon

1 cup ice

¼ cup medium-hot pepper

2 tablespoons chia seed

Directions:

Combine all ingredients in a high-power blender or food processor and blend until smooth. Drink immediately.

CULINARY TIP *Choose chili peppers that have the level of heat intensity that you prefer. I like mild heat, and I love this combination of cool and hot.*

Nutrition Facts (per serving):
Calories: 100 Fat: 5 Carbs: 8 Fiber: 7 Protein: 4

AUGUST 23: MELON FREEZE

Serves 2

If you like tart and sweet, you'll love this citrusy fresh smoothie.

Ingredients:

1 cup watermelon

½ cup grapefruit

½ cup ice

2 tablespoons chia seed

1 tablespoon lime juice

Directions:

Combine all ingredients in a high-power blender or food processor and blend until smooth. Drink immediately.

Nutrition Facts (per serving):
Calories: 116 Fat: 5 Carbs: 13 Fiber: 7 Protein: 4

AUGUST 24: GINGER MELON TEA

Serves 2

The ginger root in this recipe may give you a flatter belly, as it reduces intestinal inflammation.

Ingredients:

1 cup watermelon

½ cup brewed green tea

½ cup ice

2 tablespoons fresh ginger root

2 tablespoons chia seed

1 teaspoon lime juice

Directions:

Combine all ingredients in a high-power blender
or food processor and blend until smooth.
Drink immediately.

CULINARY TIP

*Use seedless watermelon to avoid
having some of the seed pulp in
your smoothie.*

Nutrition Facts (per serving):
Calories: 97 Fat: 5 Carbs: 8 Fiber: 6 Protein: 4

AUGUST 25: WATERMELON SHAKE

Serves 2

This delicious drink is popular with kids,
as it's creamy, pink and sweet.

Ingredients:

1 cup watermelon

½ cup rice milk

½ cup nonfat Greek yogurt

½ teaspoon turmeric powder

Directions:

Combine all ingredients in a high-power blender
or food processor and blend until smooth.
Drink immediately.

Nutrition Facts (per serving):
Calories: 86 Fat: 1 Carbs: 14 Fiber: 0 Protein: 7

AUGUST 26: WATERMELON SMASH

Serves 2

This smoothie is surprisingly sweet, tasty and refreshing, with a prominent watermelon flavor. Kale is a rich source of calcium, a mineral that works with vitamin D to help us shed body fat.

Ingredients:

½ cup watermelon

½ cup ice

½ cup baby kale leaves

½ cup carrot juice

2 tablespoons chia seed

Directions:

Combine all ingredients in a high-power blender or food processor and blend until smooth. Drink immediately.

CULINARY TIP *Baby greens are tender and mild and blend more easily than more mature greens.*

Nutrition Facts (per serving):
Calories: 112 Fat: 5 Carbs: 11 Fiber: 7 Protein: 4

AUGUST 27: STRAWBERRY WATERMELON WITH CITRUS

Serves 2

Berries and melon pair well in this recipe, and a little citrus addition is sublime! Both the strawberries and watermelon are rich in vitamin C and carotenoids.

Ingredients:

½ cup frozen strawberries

½ cup water

½ cup watermelon

¼ cup ice

2 tablespoons hulled hemp seed

1 teaspoon lemon juice

Directions:

Combine all ingredients in a high-power blender
or food processor and blend until smooth.
Drink immediately.

CULINARY TIP

Use frozen watermelon and eliminate the ice for a richer flavor.

Nutrition Facts (per serving):
Calories: 69 Fat: 3 Carbs: 8 Fiber: 2 Protein: 3

AUGUST 28: WATERMELON MINT

Serves 2

Watermelon and mint pair perfectly together in
this smoothie, which contains water and ice to counter
the damaging effect of dehydration, the most common
cause of fatigue.

Ingredients:

1 cup watermelon

½ cup water

½ cup ice

½ cup frozen peaches

¼ cup fresh mint leaves

2 tablespoons chia seed

Directions:

Combine all ingredients in a high-power blender
or food processor and blend until smooth.
Drink immediately.

CULINARY TIP *Be sure to use filtered water for making ice in order to remove chlorine and other chemicals that will affect the flavor of your smoothie.*

Nutrition Facts (per serving):
Calories: 109 Fat: 5 Carbs: 11 Fiber: 7 Protein: 4

AUGUST 29: WATERMELON LIME COOLER

Serves 2

This smoothie has a predominantly watermelon flavor
with berry and citrus notes. Coconut water adds a light
coconut flavor and is rich in potassium.

Ingredients:

1 cup watermelon

1 cup coconut water

½ cup frozen strawberries

¼ cup Meyer lemon

2 tablespoons chia seed

2 tablespoons lime juice

Directions:

Combine all ingredients in a high-power blender
or food processor and blend until smooth.
Drink immediately.

Add a pinch of salt to bring out the strawberry and basil flavors.

Nutrition Facts (per serving):
Calories: 134 Fat: 5 Carbs: 18 Fiber: 8 Protein: 4

AUGUST 30: WATERMELON WITH TURMERIC

Serves 2

Sweet melon and berries flavor this drink, and bright yellow turmeric adds color and fragrance.

Ingredients:
1 cup watermelon
½ cup frozen strawberries
½ cup coconut water
2 tablespoons chia seed
½ teaspoon turmeric powder

Directions:
Combine all ingredients in a high-power blender or food processor and blend until smooth.
Drink immediately.

You can use fresh or frozen watermelon interchangeably in this smoothie.

Nutrition Facts (per serving):
Calories: 116 Fat: 5 Carbs: 13 Fiber: 7 Protein: 4

AUGUST 31: WATERMELON ORANGE POWER

Serves 2

This fresh, juicy combination is sweet with a golden glow from the turmeric and delivers a decent amount of fiber and protein!

Ingredients:

1 cup watermelon

1 cup orange

½ cup ice

2 tablespoons chia seed

2 tablespoons protein powder

½ teaspoon turmeric powder

Directions:

Combine all ingredients in a high-power blender or food processor and blend until smooth.
Drink immediately.

Nutrition Facts (per serving):
Calories: 155 Fat: 5 Carbs: 18 Fiber: 8 Protein: 8

CHAPTER 12

September Smoothies

PEACH NECTAR SMOOTHIES

SEPTEMBER 1: PEACH APRICOT NECTARINE

Serves 2

This recipe is a creamy blend that is rich in tart stone fruit flavor with a bit of citrus.

Ingredients:
1 apricot
1 nectarine
½ cup peach nectar
½ cup frozen peaches
½ cup ice
½ cup nonfat Greek yogurt
1 teaspoon lemon juice

Directions:
Combine all ingredients in a high-power blender or food processor and blend until smooth.
Drink immediately.

Nutrition Facts (per serving):
Calories: 127 Fat: 0 Carbs: 25 Fiber: 2 Protein: 8

SEPTEMBER 2: SOUTHERN BELLE

Serves 2

This variation on the classic peaches-and-cream dish is so delicious that you'll want to have it every day!

Ingredients:

½ cup peach nectar

½ cup ice

½ cup rice milk

½ cup nonfat Greek yogurt

1 pinch of ground cinnamon

Directions:

Combine all ingredients in a high-power blender or food processor and blend until smooth. Drink immediately.

CULINARY TIP *Cinnamon adds depth of flavor and an aromatic complement to the peach nectar.*

Nutrition Facts (per serving):
Calories: 98 Fat: 1 Carbs: 16 Fiber: 0 Protein: 6

ALMOND MILK SMOOTHIES

SEPTEMBER 3: COCOA CASHEW DREAM

Serves 1

This drink is creamy, rich and chocolaty.

Ingredients:

1 frozen banana

1 cup almond milk

1 tablespoon cashews

1 tablespoon unsweetened cocoa powder

Directions:

Combine all ingredients in a high-power blender or food processor and blend until smooth. Drink immediately.

Nutrition Facts (per serving):
Calories: 233 Fat: 9 Carbs: 33 Fiber: 5 Protein: 6

SEPTEMBER 4: BLUEBERRY NUTMEG

Serves 2

Creamy, subtle blueberry flavor shines in this smoothie, with a hint of nutmeg.

Ingredients:

½ frozen banana

½ cup almond milk

½ cup nonfat Greek yogurt

½ cup frozen wild blueberries

1 pinch of fresh ground nutmeg

Directions:

Combine all ingredients in a high-power blender or food processor and blend until smooth. Drink immediately.

CULINARY **TIP** *Avoid the flavored milk alternatives, such as chocolate almond milk, as they have a higher sugar content.*

Nutrition Facts (per serving):
Calories: 84 Fat: 1 Carbs: 14 Fiber: 2 Protein: 7

SEPTEMBER 5: ALMOND DATE COFFEE

Serves 1

This is a light and refreshing pick-me-up for the
morning or for an afternoon wake-up from a nap.
It is also a very low-calorie way to get a caffeine boost.

Ingredients:

1 Medjool date
½ cup almond milk
½ cup ice
1 tablespoon chia seed
1 teaspoon instant coffee

Directions:

Combine all ingredients in a high-power blender
or food processor and blend until smooth.
Drink immediately.

CULINARY **TIP** *Add ½ a frozen banana to the smoothie for a creamier texture.*

Nutrition Facts (per serving):
Calories: 151 Fat: 6 Carbs: 19 Fiber: 8 Protein: 4

SEPTEMBER 6: SWEET ALMOND CREAM

Serves 1

This creamy treat is smooth with a strong nutmeg
flavor and scent.

Ingredients:

½ cup almond milk
½ cup frozen cherries
½ cup nonfat Greek yogurt
1 teaspoon vanilla extract
1 pinch of fresh ground nutmeg

Directions:

Combine all ingredients in a high-power blender
or food processor and blend until smooth.
Drink immediately.

Nutrition Facts (per serving):
Calories: 142 Fat: 1 Carbs: 18 Fiber: 2 Protein: 13

SEPTEMBER 7: CREAMY ALMOND DATE

Serves 2

A toasted almond flavor combines with creamy yogurt
in this protein-rich drink that is just a little sweet.
Studies have found that a higher protein diet equates
to a higher rate of weight loss.

Ingredients:

1 Medjool date
½ cup almond milk
½ cup ice
½ cup nonfat Greek yogurt
2 tablespoons roasted and chopped almonds

Directions:

Combine all ingredients in a high-power blender
or food processor and blend until smooth.
Drink immediately.

CULINARY TIP *One tablespoon of almond butter can be used instead of chopped almonds and will provide a creamier texture.*

Nutrition Facts (per serving):
Calories: 154 Fat: 8 Carbs: 13 Fiber: 3 Protein: 9

SEPTEMBER 8: SWEET CHERRY CREAM

Serves 2

This blend with sweet cherries is frosty and rich.

Ingredients:

½ frozen banana

½ cup almond milk

½ cup ice

½ cup frozen sweet cherries

2 tablespoons chia seed

Directions:

Combine all ingredients in a high-power blender or food processor and blend until smooth. Drink immediately.

Nutrition Facts (per serving):
Calories: 127 Fat: 6 Carbs: 14 Fiber: 8 Protein: 4

SEPTEMBER 9: LEMON VANILLA CREAM

Serves 2

Light lemon and vanilla flavors shine in this protein-rich smoothie.

Ingredients:

½ frozen banana

½ cup almond milk

½ cup ice

½ cup nonfat Greek yogurt

1 teaspoon lemon juice

½ teaspoon vanilla extract

Directions:

Combine all ingredients in a high-power blender or food processor and blend until smooth. Drink immediately.

Nutrition Facts (per serving):
Calories: 70 Fat: 1 Carbs: 9 Fiber: 1 Protein: 7

SEPTEMBER 10: ALMOND CRUNCH

Serves 2

You'll enjoy a subtle almond flavor with crunchy bits of almonds and an energy boost from this creamy smoothie. Because of the higher calorie count, consider this a meal-replacement smoothie instead of a snack.

Ingredients:

1 date

½ cup almond milk

½ cup ice

½ cup nonfat Greek yogurt

¼ cup roasted and chopped almonds

2 tablespoons hulled hemp seed

Directions:

Combine all ingredients in a high-power blender or food processor and blend until smooth. Drink immediately.

CULINARY TIP *Chopped roasted almonds are available in the bulk foods section of many grocery stores.*

Nutrition Facts (per serving):
Calories: 279 Fat: 18 Carbs: 17 Fiber: 6 Protein: 15

SEPTEMBER 11: COCONUT ALMOND COCOA

Serves 1

Chocolaty with a bit of coconut, this smoothie tastes similar to an almond-coconut chocolate bar but not too sweet. Cocoa contains flavanols, which have been shown to lower blood pressure by relaxing blood vessels.

Ingredients:
½ cup almond milk

½ cup ice

1 tablespoon roasted and chopped almonds

1 tablespoon unsweetened fine macaroon coconut

1 tablespoon unsweetened cocoa powder

Directions:
Combine all ingredients in a high-power blender or food processor and blend until smooth. Drink immediately.

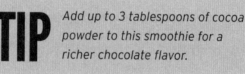

CULINARY TIP *Add up to 3 tablespoons of cocoa powder to this smoothie for a richer chocolate flavor.*

Nutrition Facts (per serving):
Calories: 147 Fat: 12 Carbs: 5 Fiber: 4 Protein: 5

SEPTEMBER 12: VANILLA CHERRY ALMOND

Serves 2

The vanilla fragrance in this recipe hits your nose before the cherry flavor pops in your mouth! Cherries are also an excellent source of fiber.

Ingredients:

½ cup almond milk

½ cup ice

½ cup frozen cherries

2 tablespoons roasted and chopped almonds

½ teaspoon vanilla extract

Directions:

Combine all ingredients in a high-power blender or food processor and blend until smooth. Drink immediately.

CULINARY TIP *Vanilla extract is made from tropical vanilla beans native to Mexico, Central America and the Caribbean.*

Nutrition Facts (per serving):
Calories: 114 Fat: 8 Carbs: 8 Fiber: 3 Protein: 4

SEPTEMBER 13: CHOCOLATE ALMOND MILKSHAKE

Serves 2

Enjoy this rich and sweet milkshake that has almond and vanilla flavor without all the guilt. Almonds help us take in the 25 grams of fiber per day shown to lower the risk for hypertension and high cholesterol.

Ingredients:

½ frozen banana

½ cup almond milk

½ cup ice

½ cup nonfat Greek yogurt

1 tablespoon unsweetened cocoa powder

1 tablespoon roasted and chopped almonds

1 teaspoon vanilla extract

Directions:

Combine all ingredients in a high-power blender
or food processor and blend until smooth.
Drink immediately.

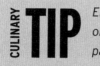

CULINARY TIP *Either buy almond milk pre-made or make fresh almond milk (see page 12).*

Nutrition Facts (per serving):
Calories: 123 Fat: 5 Carbs: 11 Fiber: 2 Protein: 9

SEPTEMBER 14: BANANA ALMOND DATE

Serves 2

This smoothie is creamy, nutty and reminiscent of
eggnog. Studies show that increasing protein intake
from dietary sources such as yogurt and nuts—like
those included in this recipe—reduces the appetite
and sugar cravings.

Ingredients:

2 Medjool dates

½ frozen banana

½ cup almond milk

½ cup nonfat Greek yogurt

¼ cup cashews

1 pinch of fresh ground nutmeg

Directions:

Combine all ingredients in a high-power blender
or food processor and blend until smooth.
Drink immediately.

CULINARY **TIP** *Yogurt and cashews provide the creamy texture and protein in this drink.*

Nutrition Facts (per serving):
Calories: 231 Fat: 8 Carbs: 33 Fiber: 3 Protein: 10

SEPTEMBER 15: VANILLA CASHEW DREAM

Serves 2

I could drink this every day. The ground cashews give this smoothie a pudding-like quality that's so delicious it could be served as a dessert! Because of the higher calorie count, consider this to be a meal-replacement smoothie instead of a snack.

Ingredients:

1 frozen banana
1 vanilla bean
½ cup almond milk
½ cup nonfat Greek yogurt
¼ cup cashews
1 tablespoon unsweetened cocoa powder

Directions:

Combine all ingredients in a high-power blender or food processor and blend until smooth. Drink immediately.

CULINARY **TIP** *Unsweetened cocoa powder is rich in antioxidants and contains no sugar. Add an extra tablespoon of cocoa if you like a richer chocolate flavor.*

Nutrition Facts (per serving):
Calories: 262 Fat: 13 Carbs: 26 Fiber: 3 Protein: 13

SEPTEMBER 16: ROASTED ALMOND SHAKE

Serves 1

Almonds provide protein, fiber and healthful fats in this creamy, nutty and rich recipe that tastes almost like a dessert.

Ingredients:

½ frozen banana

½ cup almond milk

1 tablespoon roasted and chopped almonds

Directions:

Combine all ingredients in a high-power blender or food processor and blend until smooth. Drink immediately.

CULINARY TIP *Add a few drops of almond extract for an even deeper flavor.*

Nutrition Facts (per serving):
Calories: 147 Fat: 8 Carbs: 15 Fiber: 4 Protein: 4

FRESH BLUEBERRY SMOOTHIES

SEPTEMBER 17: BERRY BLUES

Serves 2

The color in the berries of this antioxidant-rich smoothie is from health-promoting polyphenols, so the richer the color, the more antioxidants there are in the smoothie.

Ingredients:

1 cup blueberry nectar

½ cup blueberries

½ cup frozen raspberries

½ cup ice

2 tablespoons chia seed

Directions:

Combine all ingredients in a high-power blender or food processor and blend until smooth. Drink immediately.

CULINARY TIP *Frozen raspberries provide rich texture and color but can often be a bit tart. Adding some fruit juice nectar will sweeten up a smoothie.*

Nutrition Facts (per serving):
Calories: 168 Fat: 5 Carbs: 25 Fiber: 10 Protein: 3

SEPTEMBER 18: ANTIOXIDANT MAXIMIZER

Serves 2

In this smoothie, you'll find sweet blueberry flavor with tart pomegranate undertones, as well as antioxidant polyphenols that give this smoothie its deep red-purple coloring.

Ingredients:

1 cup blueberry nectar

½ cup pomegranate juice

½ cup blueberries

½ cup ice

2 tablespoons chia seed

Directions:

Combine all ingredients in a high-power blender or food processor and blend until smooth.
Drink immediately.

CULINARY TIP *Pomegranate juice is much easier to use in smoothies than pomegranate arils, as the seeds are large, and it can be hard for a blender to break them down.*

Nutrition Facts (per serving):
Calories: 186 Fat: 5 Carbs: 30 Fiber: 8 Protein: 3

SEPTEMBER 19: BLUEBERRY ALMOND

Serves 1

This smoothie is a thick, exotic blend with rich almond and date flavors. Daily consumption of whole blueberries has been proven in numerous studies to reduce the risk for diabetes, as blueberries increase insulin sensitivity. Because of the higher calorie count, consider this a meal-replacement smoothie instead of a snack.

Ingredients:
1 Medjool date
½ cup blueberries
½ cup brewed green tea
2 tablespoons roasted and chopped almonds

Directions:
Combine all ingredients in a high-power blender or food processor and blend until smooth.
Drink immediately.

Nutrition Facts (per serving):
Calories: 261 Fat: 14 Carbs: 32 Fiber: 9 Protein: 6

SEPTEMBER 20: THE VIOLET TUTU

Serves 2

The ingredients in this drink make it creamy, rich and full of fresh flavor. Blueberry phytochemicals have been found to alleviate hyperglycemia.

Ingredients:

½ frozen banana

1 cup coconut water

½ cup ice

½ cup blueberries

½ cup avocado

2 tablespoons chia seed

Directions:

Combine all ingredients in a high-power blender or food processor and blend until smooth. Drink immediately.

CULINARY TIP *Use a fresh avocado with an even green coloring and no brown spots on the flesh, as that indicates the avocado is overripe.*

Nutrition Facts (per serving):
Calories: 204 Fat: 10 Carbs: 23 Fiber: 12 Protein: 5

SEPTEMBER 21: BLUEBERRY BANANA

Serves 2

This is a tasty and creamy smoothie, with a rich blueberry flavor and a hit of protein for energy.

Ingredients:

1 frozen banana

½ cup almond milk

½ cup blueberries

½ cup ice

2 tablespoons vanilla-flavored protein powder

Directions:

Combine all ingredients in a high-power blender
or food processor and blend until smooth.
Drink immediately.

CULINARY TIP *Vanilla whey protein powders, such as Spiru-Tein by Nature's Plus, provide essential amino acids as well as a creamy texture and sweet flavor to smoothies.*

Nutrition Facts (per serving):
Calories: 100 Fat: 1 Carbs: 19 Fiber: 3 Protein: 5

FUJI APPLE SMOOTHIES

SEPTEMBER 22: CINNAMON APPLE CREAM

Serves 2

A luscious fresh apple flavor is the base in this
cinnamon treat!

Ingredients:

½ Fuji apple

½ cup oat milk

½ cup ice

½ cup nonfat Greek yogurt

¼ teaspoon cinnamon

Directions:

Combine all ingredients in a high-power blender or food processor and blend until smooth. Drink immediately.

Unsweetened applesauce (½ cup) can be used in place of the fresh apple if you're out of apples.

Nutrition Facts (per serving):
Calories: 89 Fat: 1 Carbs: 14 Fiber: 2 Protein: 7

SEPTEMBER 23: KEY LIME PIE

Serves 2

Fresh lime and banana flavors come through in this recipe, with a hint of sweet crisp Fuji apple.

Ingredients:

½ frozen banana

½ Fuji apple

½ cup coconut water

2 tablespoons lime juice

2 tablespoons hulled hemp seed

Directions:

Combine all ingredients in a high-power blender or food processor and blend until smooth. Drink immediately.

Apple and banana go together perfectly, like chocolate and vanilla.

Nutrition Facts (per serving):
Calories: 105 Fat: 3 Carbs: 17 Fiber: 3 Protein: 3

SEPTEMBER 24: CHERRY BASIL

Serves 2

This recipe combines a sweet apple flavor with sweet, fragrant, herbaceous holy basil fragrance.

Ingredients:

½ Fuji apple

½ cup black cherry juice

½ cup ice

¼ cup fresh holy basil leaves

2 tablespoons chia seed

Directions:

Combine all ingredients in a high-power blender or food processor and blend until smooth. Drink immediately.

CULINARY TIP *Fresh holy basil leaves are delicious and give smoothies an inviting scent. They also help to regulate blood sugar.*

Nutrition Facts (per serving):
Calories: 126 Fat: 5 Carbs: 15 Fiber: 7 Protein: 3

SEPTEMBER 25: FUJI MINT CRUSH

Serves 2

Apples provide flavonols that protect us from cancer and promote healthy cell development.

Ingredients:

½ Fuji apple

½ cup unfiltered apple juice

½ cup ice

½ cup nonfat Greek yogurt

¼ cup fresh mint leaves

Directions:

Combine all ingredients in a high-power blender or food processor and blend until smooth.

Drink immediately.

Nutrition Facts (per serving):
Calories: 87 Fat: 0 Carbs: 16 Fiber: 1 Protein: 6

SEPTEMBER 26: SPICED APPLE CIDER

Serves 1

Apples are an excellent source of soluble fiber, which holds onto water in our digestive tracts, allowing the water to hydrate us over many hours.

Ingredients:

½ Fuji apple

½ cup unfiltered apple juice

½ cup ice

1 tablespoon chia seed

1 pinch of cinnamon

1 pinch of cardamom

1 pinch of fresh ground black pepper

Directions:

Combine all ingredients in a high-power blender or food processor and blend until smooth.

Drink immediately.

Nutrition Facts (per serving):
Calories: 174 Fat: 5 Carbs: 28 Fiber: 8 Protein: 3

SEPTEMBER 27: MOUNTAIN BREEZE

Serves 2

This drink is bitter and tart, yet also sweet with apple flavor. Fresh juices from apples and grapefruit contain antioxidants that can protect cells from oxidative stress, thus reducing inflammation.

Ingredients:

1 Fuji apple

½ cup unfiltered apple juice

½ cup ice

½ cup grapefruit juice

2 tablespoons chia seed

Directions:

Combine all ingredients in a high-power blender or food processor and blend until smooth. Drink immediately.

CULINARY TIP *I love the flavor of Fuji apples, but all apples provide antioxidants, so choose according to your taste.*

Nutrition Facts (per serving):
Calories: 168 Fat: 5 Carbs: 26 Fiber: 8 Protein: 4

STAR FRUIT SMOOTHIES

SEPTEMBER 28: STAR FRUIT TEA

Serves 2

This delicate combination has a light mint fragrance and sweet, astringent star fruit flavor. Additionally, star fruit is a potent source of polyphenolic antioxidants.

Ingredients:

1 star fruit

1 cup brewed green tea

½ cup ice

¼ cup fresh mint leaves

2 tablespoons chia seed

Directions:

Combine all ingredients in a high-power blender or food processor and blend until smooth. Drink immediately.

CULINARY TIP

Star fruit (aka carambola) has a sweet but acidic flavor that gives smoothies an exotic flair.

Nutrition Facts (per serving):
Calories: 86 Fat: 5 Carbs: 5 Fiber: 8 Protein: 4

SEPTEMBER 29: STAR FRUIT AND CREAM

Serves 2

This smoothie is tannic and perfumed with the delightful scent of star fruit (aka carambola).

Ingredients:

1 star fruit

½ cup unfiltered apple juice

½ cup ice

½ cup nonfat Greek yogurt

Directions:

Combine all ingredients in a high-power blender or food processor and blend until smooth. Drink immediately.

Nutrition Facts (per serving):
Calories: 76 Fat: 0 Carbs: 12 Fiber: 1 Protein: 7

SEPTEMBER 30: STAR FRUIT AND PAPAYA

Serves 2

This smoothie is fresh and nutrient rich, with a citrus high note. Preliminary studies have found that just the smell of vanilla helps with weight loss by creating a sense of satiety rather than deprivation.

Ingredients:

1 star fruit

1 cup papaya

½ cup watermelon

½ cup coconut water

½ cup ice

1 teaspoon lemon juice

½ teaspoon vanilla extract

Directions:

Combine all ingredients in a high-power blender or food processor and blend until smooth. Drink immediately.

CULINARY TIP *Vanilla balances lemon and adds depth of flavor.*

Nutrition Facts (per serving):
Calories: 69 Fat: 0 Carbs: 17 Fiber: 3 Protein: 1

CHAPTER 13

October Smoothies

COCONUT WATER SMOOTHIES

OCTOBER 1: COCONUT BLACKBERRY ICY

Serves 1

This drink is slightly sweet and light, with rich berry flavor. The bananas provide an excellent source of vitamin B_6.

Ingredients:

½ frozen banana

½ cup coconut water

½ cup frozen blackberries

1 tablespoon chia seed

Directions:

Combine all ingredients in a high-power blender or food processor and blend until smooth. Drink immediately.

All berries blend well with banana and coconut water, so if you don't have blackberries on hand, you can just use whatever berries you have in your freezer.

Nutrition Facts (per serving):
Calories: 190 Fat: 4 Carbs: 37 Fiber: 11 Protein: 4

OCTOBER 2: CHOCOLATE BANANA CASHEW

Serves 2

This recipe has creamy banana and cashew flavors, with subtle cocoa tones laced throughout. The cashews are a good source of calcium, which helps fat cells release stored body fat.

Ingredients:

1 frozen banana

1 cup coconut water

½ cup ice

2 tablespoons cashews

2 tablespoons hulled hemp seed

1 tablespoon unsweetened cocoa powder

Directions:

Combine all ingredients in a high-power blender or food processor and blend until smooth. Drink immediately.

Cashew butter or even peanut butter can be used instead of whole cashews, if desired.

Nutrition Facts (per serving):
Calories: 178 Fat: 7 Carbs: 24 Fiber: 3 Protein: 5

OCTOBER 3: LEMON VANILLA DROP

Serves 2

In this smoothie, you'll taste a sour lemon flavor with a tinge of sweetness. Coconut water contains only about 60 calories per cup versus dairy milk (whole), which contains about 150 calories per cup.

Ingredients:

½ cucumber

1 cup coconut water

1 cup ice

2 tablespoons chia seed

1 tablespoon lemon juice

1 teaspoon coconut nectar

1 teaspoon vanilla extract

Directions:

Combine all ingredients in a high-power blender or food processor and blend until smooth. Drink immediately.

Nutrition Facts (per serving):
Calories: 112 Fat: 4 Carbs: 15 Fiber: 6 Protein: 3

OCTOBER 4: COCONUT COFFEE

Serves 1

This smoothie is as frosty and rich as a blended caffe latte and just as satisfying.

Ingredients:

½ frozen banana

½ cup coconut water

¼ cup ice

1 tablespoon vanilla-flavored protein powder

1 teaspoon instant coffee

¼ teaspoon vanilla extract

Directions:

Combine all ingredients in a high-power blender or food processor and blend until smooth. Drink immediately.

CULINARY TIP *For a more exotic vanilla flavor, use ½ a vanilla bean instead of vanilla extract.*

Nutrition Facts (per serving):
Calories: 98 Fat: 0 Carbs: 20 Fiber: 2 Protein: 5

OCTOBER 5: THE GOLDEN BERRY

Serves 1

This is a simple and refreshing blend. The coconut water is an excellent source of potassium, and in lab studies, phytochemicals in wild blueberries helped alleviate hyperglycemia.

Ingredients:

½ cup coconut water

½ cup ice

½ cup frozen wild blueberries

1 tablespoon chia seed

¼ teaspoon turmeric powder

1 pinch of fresh ground black pepper

Directions:

Combine all ingredients in a high-power blender or food processor and blend until smooth. Drink immediately.

If you prefer, you can leave the ice out of any smoothie recipe that includes it. It's simply there to cool the drink, create texture and add water for hydration. Without the ice, the flavors are richer and deeper.

Nutrition Facts (per serving):
Calories: 126 Fat: 5 Carbs: 16 Fiber: 9 Protein: 3

OCTOBER 6: COCONUT COFFEE MOCHA

Serves 1

Wake up with this drink that includes your favorite coffee flavors and a solid dose of vegan protein for hours of nutrient-supported energy.

Ingredients:

½ frozen banana

½ cup coconut water

2 tablespoons hulled hemp seed

1 tablespoon unsweetened cocoa powder

1 teaspoon instant coffee

¼ teaspoon vanilla extract

Directions:

Combine all ingredients in a high-power blender or food processor and blend until smooth. Drink immediately.

Instant coffee is almost as rich in antioxidants as brewed coffee.

Nutrition Facts (per serving):
Calories: 186 Fat: 7 Carbs: 24 Fiber: 5 Protein: 7

OCTOBER 7: ALMOND COCOA COCONUT CRUNCH

Serves 1

This smoothie is rich in healthful fats that moisturize the skin and give hair its luster.

Ingredients:

½ frozen banana

1 cup coconut water

1 tablespoon roasted and chopped almonds

1 tablespoon unsweetened fine macaroon coconut

1 tablespoon unsweetened cocoa powder

Directions:

Combine all ingredients in a high-power blender or food processor and blend until smooth. Drink immediately.

Nutrition Facts (per serving):
Calories: 227 Fat: 11 Carbs: 29 Fiber: 6 Protein: 5

OCTOBER 8: BLUEBERRY VANILLA REFRESHER

Serves 1

This is a very low-calorie hydrating smoothie that is chock full of energizing electrolytes!

Ingredients:

½ cup coconut water

½ cup ice

½ cup frozen wild blueberries

1 teaspoon lemon juice

½ teaspoon vanilla extract

Directions:

Combine all ingredients in a high-power blender or food processor and blend until smooth. Drink immediately.

Nutrition Facts (per serving):
Calories: 62 Fat: 0 Carbs: 15 Fiber: 3 Protein: 0

OCTOBER 9: CHOCOLATE ALMOND DATE COCONUT

Serves 1

The unsweetened cocoa powder contains compounds that help reduce inflammation in the intestine, which lets you show off your six-pack! With the higher calorie count, you can consider this to be a meal-replacement smoothie instead of a snack.

Ingredients:

2 Medjool dates

½ cup coconut water

½ cup ice

2 tablespoons roasted and chopped almonds

1 tablespoon protein powder

2 teaspoons unsweetened cocoa powder

Directions:

Combine all ingredients in a high-power blender or food processor and blend until smooth. Drink immediately.

Nutrition Facts (per serving):
Calories: 348 Fat: 15 Carbs: 47 Fiber: 8 Protein: 12

BREWED GREEN TEA SMOOTHIES

OCTOBER 10: GREEN TEA, GINGER AND BLOOD ORANGE

Serves 2

This smoothie is cool and fresh with a strong ginger hit. Sparkling waters such as San Pellegrino and Perrier are mineral waters that help us hydrate.

Ingredients:

1 blood orange

1 cup brewed green tea

¼ cup ice

2 tablespoons chia seed

1 tablespoon fresh ginger root

1 cup sparkling water

Directions:

Combine blood orange, green tea, ice, chia seed and ginger root in a high-power blender or food processor and blend until smooth. Then, stir in the sparkling water and drink immediately.

CULINARY TIP Add sparkling water after blending the rest of the smoothie ingredients. Then, stir just a second; otherwise, the bubbles get flattened. Sparkling water adds a nice effect to smoothies and it is worth perfecting the technique.

Nutrition Facts (per serving):
Calories: 106 Fat: 5 Carbs: 10 Fiber: 8 Protein: 4

OCTOBER 11: TANGY AND SWEET

Serves 2

In this frosty combination, you'll taste the earthy green tea flavor, sweet pineapple and blueberry, with a bit of tart kiwi.

Ingredients:

1 kiwi

1 cup brewed green tea

½ cup frozen wild blueberries

½ cup frozen pineapple

2 tablespoons chia seed

Directions:

Combine all ingredients in a high-power blender or food processor and blend until smooth. Drink immediately.

CULINARY TIP *Intensely sweet fruits, such as pineapple and wild blueberries, pair well with the herbal flavor of green tea.*

Nutrition Facts (per serving):
Calories: 129 Fat: 5 Carbs: 16 Fiber: 9 Protein: 4

OCTOBER 12: VIOLET TEA ELIXIR

Serves 2

Hot, fresh ginger is the highlight of this sweet, tea-based smoothie. This combo provides a triple hit of antioxidants, as the apple contains quercetin, the wild blueberries are a rich source of polyphenols and the green tea is infused with flavonoids.

Ingredients:

½ apple

1 cup brewed green tea

½ cup frozen wild blueberries

¼ cup ice

2 tablespoons chia seed

1 tablespoon fresh ginger root

....

Directions:

Combine all ingredients in a high-power blender
or food processor and blend until smooth.
Drink immediately.

CULINARY TIP *Fresh ginger root has a strong
flavor and a pungent scent, or
for a more subtle ginger accent,
try 1 teaspoon of dried powdered ginger instead.*

Nutrition Facts (per serving):
Calories: 113 Fat: 5 Carbs: 13 Fiber: 9 Protein: 3

OCTOBER 13: SPICED ICED TEA

Serves 2

....

This smoothie is easy to drink for quick hydration,
with light cinnamon and ginger flavors. Researchers
have found that ginger may help reduce the risk of
tissue damage caused by diabetes, such as cataracts.

....

Ingredients:

½ frozen banana

1 cup brewed green tea

½ cup ice

2 tablespoons chia seed

1 tablespoon fresh ginger root

½ teaspoon ground cinnamon

Directions:

Combine all ingredients in a high-power blender or food processor and blend until smooth. Drink immediately.

CULINARY TIP
When shopping for bananas for your smoothies, look for bananas that are yellow, not green, and not overripe or brown.

Nutrition Facts (per serving):
Calories: 98 Fat: 5 Carbs: 8 Fiber: 7 Protein: 3

OCTOBER 14: CHIA ENERGY BOOSTER

Serves 2

This recipe combines raspberry and vanilla flavors sweetened with a date.

Ingredients:

1 Medjool date

1 cup brewed green tea

½ cup frozen raspberries

½ cup ice

2 tablespoons chia seed

1 teaspoon acacia fiber

½ teaspoon vanilla extract

Directions:

Combine all ingredients in a high-power blender or food processor and blend until smooth. Drink immediately.

CULINARY **TIP** *Powdered soluble fiber supplements, such as Heather's Tummy Fiber (acacia), dissolve completely* in cold drinks. You won't even know the supplement is in there.

Nutrition Facts (per serving):
Calories: 126 Fat: 5 Carbs: 15 Fiber: 10 Protein: 4

OCTOBER 15: SOUR BERRY BREW

Serves 2

Raspberries pair well with the earthy flavor of green tea in this smoothie.

Ingredients:

1 cup brewed green tea

½ cup ice

½ cup frozen raspberries

2 tablespoons chia seed

Directions:

Combine all ingredients in a high-power blender or food processor and blend until smooth. Drink immediately.

CULINARY **TIP** *Fresh and frozen raspberries work equally well in this combination.*

Nutrition Facts (per serving):
Calories: 85 Fat: 5 Carbs: 5 Fiber: 8 Protein: 3

ORANGE JUICE SMOOTHIES

OCTOBER 16: VANILLA BEAN CREAM CITRUS

Serves 2

This smoothie tastes like an orange cream with
a little tart grapefruit.

Ingredients:

½ cup orange juice

½ cup ice

½ cup nonfat Greek yogurt

¼ cup grapefruit juice

½ teaspoon vanilla extract

Directions:

Combine all ingredients in a high-power blender
or food processor and blend until smooth.
Drink immediately.

CULINARY TIP *Use ½ a cup of fresh orange
segments instead of grapefruit
juice if you prefer a sweeter
and less tart smoothie.*

Nutrition Facts (per serving):
Calories: 75 Fat: 0 Carbs: 12 Fiber: 0 Protein: 7

OCTOBER 17: ÜBER ORANGE CITRUS

Serves 1

You'll taste layers of orange flavor in this smoothie,
with golden turmeric and tangerine.

Ingredients:

1 tangerine

½ cup ice

½ cup orange juice

1 tablespoon chia seed

1 teaspoon lime juice

¼ teaspoon turmeric powder

Directions:

Combine all ingredients in a high-power blender
or food processor and blend until smooth.
Drink immediately.

Nutrition Facts (per serving):

Calories: 165 Fat: 5 Carbs: 24 Fiber: 8 Protein: 4

OCTOBER 18: SPICED CHERRY CITRUS

Serves 1

This citrus-based fat burner is cool and invigorating
with a bit of warm spice. Fortified orange juice is an
excellent source of vitamin D, which reduces hunger
signaled by the hormone leptin.

Ingredients:

½ cup orange juice

½ cup frozen cherries

1 teaspoon lemon juice

1 pinch of ground cinnamon

1 pinch of fresh ground black pepper

Directions:

Combine all ingredients in a high-power blender
or food processor and blend until smooth.
Drink immediately.

CULINARY TIP *Add yogurt, hemp seed or protein powder to smoothies to turn them into a meal replacement.*

Nutrition Facts (per serving):

Calories: 103 Fat: 0 Carbs: 25 Fiber: 2 Protein: 2

OCTOBER 19: SPICY ORANGE CHERRY

Serves 2

This smoothie features orange and cherry flavors with the heat of ginger.

Ingredients:

½ cup orange juice

½ cup ice

½ cup frozen cherries

½ cup nonfat Greek yogurt

1 teaspoon fresh ginger root

½ teaspoon turmeric powder

Directions:

Combine all ingredients in a high-power blender or food processor and blend until smooth. Drink immediately.

Nutrition Facts (per serving):
Calories: 85 Fat: 0 Carbs: 15 Fiber: 1 Protein: 7

OCTOBER 20: STRAWBERRY CITRUS

Serves 1

Sweet strawberries and tart citrus flavors are featured in this recipe. Strawberries contain powerful polyphenol compounds that reduce inflammation and water weight.

Ingredients:

½ cup frozen strawberries

½ cup orange juice

1 tablespoon hulled hemp seed

1 teaspoon lemon juice

Directions:

Combine all ingredients in a high-power blender
or food processor and blend until smooth.
Drink immediately.

CULINARY TIP *Wild strawberries are much
sweeter than cultivated berries.
Try wild strawberries, if you
can find them, for a real treat.*

Nutrition Facts (per serving):
Calories: 126 Fat: 3 Carbs: 21 Fiber: 3 Protein: 4

OCTOBER 21: CITRUS MELON

Serves 1

The lemon carries this smoothie and brightens the
orange and melon flavors.

Ingredients:

½ cup honeydew melon

½ cup ice

½ cup orange juice

1 tablespoon hulled hemp seed

1 teaspoon lemon juice

Directions:

Combine all ingredients in a high-power blender
or food processor and blend until smooth.
Drink immediately.

Nutrition Facts (per serving):
Calories: 130 Fat: 3 Carbs: 22 Fiber: 2 Protein: 4

OCTOBER 22: VANILLA ORANGE CREAM

Serves 2

This bright orange smoothie is creamy with a trace of vanilla.

Ingredients:

½ cup orange juice

½ cup ice

½ cup nonfat Greek yogurt

2 tablespoons whey protein

½ teaspoon vanilla extract

½ teaspoon turmeric powder

Directions:

Combine all ingredients in a high-power blender or food processor and blend until smooth. Drink immediately.

Nutrition Facts (per serving):
Calories: 86 Fat: 0 Carbs: 9 Fiber: 0 Protein: 11

OCTOBER 23: ANISE MANDARIN

Serves 2

This sweet Mandarin orange smoothie has a touch of licorice spice. Warming spices help stimulate digestion, waking up your metabolism.

Ingredients:

1 Mandarin orange

½ cup orange juice

½ cup ice

2 tablespoons hulled hemp seed

¼ teaspoon ground star anise

Directions:
Combine all ingredients in a high-power blender or food processor and blend until smooth. Drink immediately.

CULINARY TIP

Several alternate ingredients can be used in this smoothie, such as orange instead of Mandarin, cinnamon instead of star anise or protein powder instead of hemp.

Nutrition Facts (per serving):
Calories: 92 Fat: 3 Carbs: 13 Fiber: 2 Protein: 3

OCTOBER 24: ORANGE VANILLA LIME

Serves 1

The flavor of this smoothie is reminiscent of the creamy orange drinks of my childhood. Organisms in yogurt, such as lactobacillus and acidophilus, increase the absorption of nutrients and alleviate symptoms of lactose intolerance.

Ingredients:
1 vanilla bean
½ cup orange juice
½ cup ice
½ cup nonfat Greek yogurt
1 tablespoon lime juice

Directions:
Combine all ingredients in a high-power blender or food processor and blend until smooth. Drink immediately.

CULINARY TIP

Vanilla is key to the nostalgic flavor of this smoothie. You can increase the vanilla flavor by adding a few drops of vanilla extract.

Nutrition Facts (per serving):
Calories: 122 Fat: 0 Carbs: 18 Fiber: 0 Protein: 13

OCTOBER 25: CHOCOLATE ORANGE CREAM

Serves 2

Try this creamy orange whip with a little cocoa undertone as a snack or a dessert.

Ingredients:

½ cup orange juice

½ cup ice

½ cup hemp milk

½ cup nonfat Greek yogurt

1 tablespoon unsweetened cocoa powder

Directions:

Combine all ingredients in a high-power blender or food processor and blend until smooth. Drink immediately.

Nutrition Facts (per serving):
Calories: 106 Fat: 2 Carbs: 15 Fiber: 1 Protein: 8

HERBAL TEA SMOOTHIE

OCTOBER 26: BENGAL TIGER

Serves 2

Move over chai! Cinnamon accents this yogurt-spice tea blend. Herbal teas provide flavor without calories as the liquid base for smoothies.

Ingredients:

1 frozen banana

1 cup brewed Celestial Seasonings Bengal Spice tea

½ cup nonfat Greek yogurt

½ cup ice

1 pinch of ground cinnamon

1 pinch of fresh ground nutmeg

Directions:

Combine all ingredients in a high-power blender or food processor and blend until smooth. Drink immediately.

CULINARY TIP *Nutmeg's complex flavors come from its oils. Some varieties contain over 50 different compounds. Bengal Spice tea is an herbal tea blend from Celestial Seasonings and is available in most grocery stores.*

Nutrition Facts (per serving):
Calories: 86 Fat: 0 Carbs: 16 Fiber: 2 Protein: 7

SQUASH SMOOTHIES

OCTOBER 27: HOTACADA

Serves 2

Squash is an excellent source of fiber and mixed carotenoids.

Ingredients:

½ cucumber

½ medium-hot pepper

½ cup brewed green tea

½ cup cooked squash

¼ cup avocado

2 tablespoons chia seed

Directions:

Combine all ingredients in a high-power blender or food processor and blend until smooth.

Drink immediately.

....

Nutrition Facts (per serving):
Calories: 134 Fat: 8 Carbs: 10 Fiber: 9 Protein: 5

OCTOBER 28: BLUEBERRY PIE

Serves 1

....

Taste real blueberry pie flavor in this satisfying and hearty smoothie.

....

Ingredients:

½ cup water

½ cup frozen wild blueberries

½ cup cooked squash

½ teaspoon cinnamon

½ teaspoon lemon juice

....

Directions:

Combine all ingredients in a high-power blender or food processor and blend until smooth.

Drink immediately.

....

Nutrition Facts (per serving):
Calories: 53 Fat: 0 Carbs: 14 Fiber: 4 Protein: 1

OCTOBER 29: SWEET SQUASH

Serves 1

....

This smoothie is a squash lover's simple pleasure. Squash doesn't contain any fat or cholesterol. It is rich in electrolytes and low in calories.

....

Ingredients:

2 Medjool dates

½ cup coconut water

½ cup cooked squash

1 tablespoon chia seed

Directions:

Combine all ingredients in a high-power blender
or food processor and blend until smooth.
Drink immediately.

CULINARY TIP *Coconut water provides a slightly sweet base and a light coconut flavor for smoothies.*

Nutrition Facts (per serving):
Calories: 241 Fat: 5 Carbs: 46 Fiber: 10 Protein: 5

OCTOBER 30: TANGERINE SQUASH

Serves 2

This sweet and savory squash smoothie has a little
citrus character.

Ingredients:

½ cup cooked squash

½ cup tangerine juice

½ cup water

½ cup ice

1 tablespoon chia seed

1 teaspoon lemon juice

1 pinch of ground cinnamon

Directions:

Combine all ingredients in a high-power blender
or food processor and blend until smooth.
Drink immediately.

CULINARY TIP

There are different kinds of winter squash, such as acorn, delicata and butternut. You can use whichever variety you like the best in your squash smoothie recipes.

Nutrition Facts (per serving):
Calories: 70 Fat: 3 Carbs: 9 Fiber: 4 Protein: 2

OCTOBER 31: WINTER GARDEN

Serves 2

Tomato and squash flavors dominate this recipe with a little lime.

Ingredients:

1 tomato

½ cucumber

½ cup water

¼ cup cooked squash

1 tablespoon lime juice

1 tablespoon chia seed

½ teaspoon turmeric powder

Directions:

Combine all ingredients in a high-power blender or food processor and blend until smooth.

Drink immediately.

Nutrition Facts (per serving):
Calories: 56 Fat: 3 Carbs: 5 Fiber: 4 Protein: 3

CHAPTER 14

November Smoothies

CRANBERRY JUICE SMOOTHIES

NOVEMBER 1: APPLE CRANBERRY FREEZE

Serves 2

This jazzy, tart, spicy and sour combo has intense cranberry flavor! Xylitol is sweet and inhibits the growth of a common bacteria that causes ear infections and tooth cavities.

Ingredients:

½ cup unfiltered apple juice

½ cup ice

¼ cup cranberry juice

2 tablespoons chia seed

1 teaspoon fresh ginger root

1 teaspoon lemon juice

1 teaspoon xylitol

Directions:

Combine all ingredients in a high-power blender or food processor and blend until smooth. Drink immediately.

CULINARY TIP *Xylitol is a low-calorie powdered sweetener that dissolves well in smoothies.*

Nutrition Facts (per serving):
Calories: 113 Fat: 5 Carbs: 12 Fiber: 6 Protein: 3

NOVEMBER 2: WATERMELON SLUSHY

Serves 2

This smoothie is cool, fresh, tart and flavorful. The orange extract adds flavor without adding sugar or calories.

Ingredients:

1 cup watermelon

½ cup cranberry juice

½ cup black cherry juice

2 tablespoons chia seed

1 teaspoon orange extract

Directions:

Combine all ingredients in a high-power blender or food processor and blend until smooth. Drink immediately.

CULINARY TIP *When seedless watermelon is available, prep it for freezing so you'll have some on hand for months. Simply remove the rind, cut into chunks, and freeze in a wax paper or plastic food storage bag.*

Nutrition Facts (per serving):
Calories: 154 Fat: 5 Carbs: 22 Fiber: 6 Protein: 4

NOVEMBER 3: APPLE CRANBERRY ORANGE

Serves 2

The tartness of cranberry juice is balanced with sweet fruit flavors in this classic blend.

Ingredients:

1 Fuji apple

1 frozen banana

½ cup orange juice

¼ cup cranberry juice

2 tablespoons hulled hemp seed

Directions:

Combine all ingredients in a high-power blender or food processor and blend until smooth. Drink immediately.

CULINARY TIP *If the cranberry juice is too tart for your taste, substitute with orange juice.*

Nutrition Facts (per serving):
Calories: 186 Fat: 3 Carbs: 38 Fiber: 5 Protein: 4

FRESH GINGER ROOT SMOOTHIES

NOVEMBER 4: STRAWBERRY LIME GINGER

Serves 1

This smoothie has a lightly sweet green tea base with a little citrus and ginger flavor.

Ingredients:

1 cup frozen strawberries

1 cup brewed green tea

½ cup ice

2 tablespoons fresh ginger root

2 tablespoons chia seed

1 teaspoon lime juice

Directions:

Combine all ingredients in a high-power blender
or food processor and blend until smooth.
Drink immediately.

Nutrition Facts (per serving):
Calories: 100 Fat: 5 Carbs: 9 Fiber: 8 Protein: 3

NOVEMBER 5: GINGER POM

Serves 1

Enjoy Far East flavors in this smoothie, rich in weight-
loss nutrients. Also included in this smoothie are
pomegranate seeds, a potent source of antioxidants.

Ingredients:

1 cup coconut water

½ cup frozen pomegranate seeds

¼ cup fresh mint leaves

2 teaspoons fresh ginger root

Directions:

Combine all ingredients in a high-power blender
or food processor and blend until smooth.
Drink immediately.

CULINARY TIP *Use ½ a cup of pomegranate juice instead of pomegranate seeds if you prefer your smoothies without the seed fiber.*

Nutrition Facts (per serving):
Calories: 122 Fat: 0 Carbs: 29 Fiber: 4 Protein: 2

NOVEMBER 6: GINGER LIME COOLER

Serves 2

This spicy version of limeade is ultra refreshing with sparkling water. The ginger is a mild anti-inflammatory and provides antioxidants that support the immune system.

Ingredients:

2 cups sparkling water

1 cup ice

½ lime

1 teaspoon fresh ginger root

1 teaspoon coconut palm nectar

Directions:

Combine just 1 cup of sparkling water, ice, lime, ginger and coconut palm nectar in a high-power blender or food processor and blend until smooth. Then, stir in the second cup of sparkling water and drink immediately.

CULINARY TIP *Both lemon and lime complement the ginger flavor.*

Nutrition Facts (per serving):
Calories: 24 Fat: 0 Carbs: 7 Fiber: 2 Protein: 1

NOVEMBER 7: GINGER TEA SPRITZER

Serves 2

This drink is slushy, light and bubbly, with a tang of ginger heat. Many sparkling waters, such as San Pellegrino, are carbonated with carbon dioxide, which has no negative health effects versus unhealthy phosphoric acid, which is used to carbonate most sodas.

Ingredients:

1 cup brewed green tea
½ cup ice
2 tablespoons fresh ginger root
½ cup sparkling water

Directions:

Combine the green tea, ice and ginger in a high-power blender or food processor and blend until smooth. Then, stir in the sparkling water and drink immediately.

Nutrition Facts (per serving):
Calories: 4 Fat: 0 Carbs: 1 Fiber: 0 Protein: 0

PAPAYA NECTAR SMOOTHIES

NOVEMBER 8: STRAWBERRY MANGO FROSTY

Serves 2

Cold and thirst quenching, this simple smoothie is equally as appropriate as an afternoon pick-me-up or a light dessert. Strawberries are sweet but low in glycemic load, as they are rich in soluble fiber.

Ingredients:

1 cup papaya nectar
½ cup frozen strawberries
½ cup frozen mango
½ cup ice
2 tablespoons chia seed

Directions:

Combine all ingredients in a high-power blender or food processor and blend until smooth. Drink immediately.

CULINARY TIP *Either fresh or frozen fruits can be used in any smoothie recipe. Frozen fruits are often preferred, as they create a thick, milkshake-like texture when blended.*

Nutrition Facts (per serving):
Calories: 172 Fat: 5 Carbs: 26 Fiber: 7 Protein: 4

NOVEMBER 9: TROPICAL WHIP

Serves 2

The ingredients in this smoothie provide a protein-rich, creamy, tropical blend.

Ingredients:

½ frozen banana

½ cup papaya nectar

½ cup frozen mango

½ cup ice

½ cup nonfat Greek yogurt

Directions:

Combine all ingredients in a high-power blender
or food processor and blend until smooth.
Drink immediately.

Nutrition Facts (per serving):
Calories: 116 Fat: 0 Carbs: 23 Fiber: 1 Protein: 7

NOVEMBER 10: PAPAYA COOLER

Serves 2

This simple blend is sweet and light and has
a tropical fragrance.

Ingredients:

½ cup brewed green tea

½ cup ice

½ cup papaya nectar

¼ cup papaya

2 tablespoons chia seed

½ teaspoon turmeric powder

Directions:

Combine all ingredients in a high-power blender
or food processor and blend until smooth.
Drink immediately.

Nutrition Facts (per serving):
Calories: 110 Fat: 5 Carbs: 11 Fiber: 6 Protein: 3

RICE MILK SMOOTHIES

NOVEMBER 11: FIVE SPICE COCONUT

Serves 2

You'll taste a frosty blend of spice and sweetness in this smoothie. With the higher calorie count, you can consider this to be a meal-replacement smoothie instead of a snack. If you find yourself eating dinner late, you might consider trying a "meal replacement" smoothie which will metabolize more quickly than a meal, allowing more restful sleep.

Ingredients:

½ frozen banana

½ cup rice milk

½ cup coconut water

½ cup ice

2 tablespoons chia seed

2 tablespoons coconut oil

1 pinch of five-spice powder

Directions:

Combine all ingredients in a high-power blender or food processor and blend until smooth.
Drink immediately.

CULINARY TIP Five-spice powder is a common Chinese spice that contains cloves, cardamom, star anise, Sichuan pepper and fennel. Cloves contain antioxidant polyphenols that have shown promise as a protector against ultraviolet-induced skin cancer.

Nutrition Facts (per serving):
Calories: 266 Fat: 20 Carbs: 16 Fiber: 7 Protein: 4

NOVEMBER 12: CHERRY VANILLA CREAM

Serves 2

This fragrant vanilla combination works equally well as a breakfast drink or a dessert.

Ingredients:

1 cup rice milk

½ cup frozen cherries

½ cup nonfat Greek yogurt

½ cup ice

½ teaspoon vanilla extract

Directions:

Combine all ingredients in a high-power blender or food processor and blend until smooth. Drink immediately.

Nutrition Facts (per serving):
Calories: 120 Fat: 1 Carbs: 20 Fiber: 1 Protein: 7

NOVEMBER 13: MEXICAN CHOCOLATE

Serves 1

This rich and spicy chocolate shake has a cool bite and hot undertones. Cocoa not only tastes great but it also helps regulate blood pressure.

Ingredients:

½ cup rice milk

½ cup ice

½ cup nonfat Greek yogurt

1 tablespoon vanilla-flavored protein powder

1 teaspoon unsweetened cocoa powder

1 pinch of cayenne pepper

1 pinch of ground cinnamon

Directions:

Combine all ingredients in a high-power blender or food processor and blend until smooth. Drink immediately.

CULINARY TIP

Add 2 teaspoons of instant coffee granules if you want a caffeine kick in your Mexican chocolate treat.

Nutrition Facts (per serving):
Calories: 155 Fat: 2 Carbs: 17 Fiber: 0 Protein: 17

NOVEMBER 14: GINGER BANANA CREAM

Serves 1

Enjoy this creamy banana blend with warm ginger undertones and bright golden turmeric color and fragrance.

Ingredients:

½ frozen banana

½ cup rice milk

½ cup ice

1 tablespoon chia seed

2 teaspoons fresh ginger root

¼ teaspoon turmeric powder

Directions:

Combine all ingredients in a high-power blender or food processor and blend until smooth. Drink immediately.

Nutrition Facts (per serving):
Calories: 185 Fat: 6 Carbs: 27 Fiber: 8 Protein: 4

NOVEMBER 15: CINNAMON SWIRL

Serves 1

This smoothie is simple and sweet with a pleasant tinge of cinnamon spice. According to a recent review, cinnamon may help lower cholesterol and triglycerides as well as help the body use insulin more efficiently.

Ingredients:

½ cup rice milk

½ cup ice

1 tablespoon vanilla-flavored protein powder

¼ teaspoon cinnamon

Directions:

Combine all ingredients in a high-power blender or food processor and blend until smooth. Drink immediately.

 CULINARY TIP *Add more cinnamon if you want to spice up this smoothie even more.*

Nutrition Facts (per serving):
Calories: 82 Fat: 2 Carbs: 12 Fiber: 0 Protein: 5

NOVEMBER 16: VANILLA RICE CREAM

Serves 2

This rice milk drink is creamy with subdued vanilla and banana flavors. Bananas are a good source of tryptophan, a precursor to serotonin, a brain chemical that helps regulate mood.

Ingredients:

1 frozen banana

1 cup ice

½ cup rice milk

2 tablespoons chia seed

1 teaspoon vanilla extract

Directions:

Combine all ingredients in a high-power blender or food processor and blend until smooth. Drink immediately.

Nutrition Facts (per serving):
Calories: 158 Fat: 6 Carbs: 20 Fiber: 8 Protein: 4

NOVEMBER 17: CREAMY SWEET COCOA

Serves 2

This smoothie offers chocolaty goodness with just a little kick of sweetness. Dates are nutritional powerhouses rich in fiber, potassium, B vitamins, calcium, magnesium, lutein and beta-carotene.

Ingredients:

2 Medjool dates

1 frozen banana

½ cup rice milk

½ cup ice

2 tablespoons vanilla-flavored protein powder

2 tablespoons unsweetened cocoa powder

Directions:

Combine all ingredients in a high-power blender or food processor and blend until smooth. Drink immediately.

Nutrition Facts (per serving):
Calories: 191 Fat: 2 Carbs: 40 Fiber: 4 Protein: 7

NOVEMBER 18: VANILLA CREAM COCOA

Serves 2

This comforting smoothie tastes like a creamy chocolate milkshake.

Ingredients:

½ frozen banana

½ cup rice milk

½ cup nonfat Greek yogurt

1 tablespoon unsweetened cocoa powder

½ teaspoon vanilla extract

Directions:

Combine all ingredients in a high-power blender or food processor and blend until smooth. Drink immediately.

Nutrition Facts (per serving):
Calories: 102 Fat: 1 Carbs: 16 Fiber: 1 Protein: 7

NOVEMBER 19: CARAMEL CREAM

Serves 1

This smoothie tastes like a vanilla wafer cookie.

Ingredients:

½ frozen banana

½ cup rice milk

½ cup nonfat Greek yogurt

1 tablespoon vanilla-flavored protein powder

1 teaspoon vanilla extract

1 teaspoon coconut palm nectar

Directions:

Combine all ingredients in a high-power blender or food processor and blend until smooth. Drink immediately.

CULINARY TIP *Add a pinch of cinnamon or nutmeg if you like a little spice.*

Nutrition Facts (per serving):
Calories: 231 Fat: 2 Carbs: 35 Fiber: 2 Protein: 17

NOVEMBER 20: CALLIOPE

Serves 2

This drink is poetry in a glass. Oligofructose or oligosaccharides are a form of fiber naturally found in bananas that acts as a prebiotic to help foster the growth of healthful bacteria in the gut.

Ingredients:

½ frozen banana

1 cup rice milk

½ cup frozen wild blueberries

½ cup nonfat Greek yogurt

Directions:

Combine all ingredients in a high-power blender or food processor and blend until smooth. Drink immediately.

CULINARY TIP *The banana, blueberries and yogurt provide so much flavor that water can be used in place of rice milk and it's still a rich treat.*

Nutrition Facts (per serving):
Calories: 137 Fat: 1 Carbs: 25 Fiber: 1 Protein: 7

NOVEMBER 21: VANILLA CREAM

Serves 2

This creamy drink is lightly sweet with a heady vanilla aroma.

Ingredients:

½ frozen banana

½ cup rice milk

½ cup nonfat Greek yogurt

½ teaspoon vanilla extract

Directions:

Combine all ingredients in a high-power blender or food processor and blend until smooth. Drink immediately.

Nutrition Facts (per serving):
Calories: 92 Fat: 1 Carbs: 15 Fiber: 1 Protein: 7

NOVEMBER 22: SPICED CREAM

Serves 2

This smoothie is creamy and rich like a dessert. You get double hits of protein from the yogurt and the vanilla-flavored protein powder.

Ingredients:

2 prunes

½ cup ice

½ cup rice milk

½ cup nonfat Greek yogurt

1 tablespoon vanilla-flavored protein powder

1 pinch of ground cinnamon

1 pinch of fresh ground nutmeg

Directions:

Combine all ingredients in a high-power blender
or food processor and blend until smooth.
Drink immediately.

CULINARY TIP

*Prunes add sweetness to the
yogurt, and the ground nutmeg
gives a fresh flavor and scent.*

Nutrition Facts (per serving):
Calories: 97 Fat: 1 Carbs: 15 Fiber: 1 Protein: 9

NOVEMBER 23: VANILLA ORANGE

Serves 2

This smoothie combines creamy vanilla with a touch
of orange flavor.

Ingredients:

½ cup rice milk

½ cup ice

½ cup nonfat Greek yogurt

½ cup orange juice

1 teaspoon vanilla extract

Directions:

Combine all ingredients in a high-power blender
or food processor and blend until smooth.
Drink immediately.

CULINARY TIP

*Vanilla bean can add a whole new
flavor dimension to this combination.
Use a whole vanilla bean in place of
the vanilla extract for a more complex, tasty treat.*

Nutrition Facts (per serving):
Calories: 97 Fat: 1 Carbs: 15 Fiber: 0 Protein: 7

NOVEMBER 24: HELPFUL HELEN

Serves 2

This shake is creamy, delicious and full of protein. Greek yogurt is so rich in protein that just ½ a cup (used in this smoothie) contains more protein than most protein bars.

Ingredients:

½ cup rice milk

½ cup frozen cherries

½ cup nonfat Greek yogurt

1 tablespoon protein powder

Directions:

Combine all ingredients in a high-power blender or food processor and blend until smooth. Drink immediately.

CULINARY TIP *Turmeric works well in this smoothie. Add 1 teaspoon to boost the anti-inflammatory action.*

Nutrition Facts (per serving):
Calories: 98 Fat: 1 Carbs: 15 Fiber: 1 Protein: 9

NOVEMBER 25: VANILLA RICE DREAM

Serves 2

I love this rich, nutmeg-spiced smoothie that tastes a lot like eggnog! The American diet overuses fat, sugar and salt to flavor food, while healthier cuisines depend on herbs and spices—like the ones used in this recipe—that also provide medicinal benefits.

Ingredients:

1 frozen banana

1 cup ice

½ cup rice milk

2 tablespoons vanilla-flavored protein powder

1 teaspoon vanilla extract

1 pinch of ground nutmeg

Directions:

Combine all ingredients in a high-power blender or food processor and blend until smooth. Drink immediately.

CULINARY TIP *Flavor depends largely on your protein powder. I use a vanilla-flavored whey-based powder. If yours is bitter, add a little vanilla extract to compensate.*

Nutrition Facts (per serving):
Calories: 111 Fat: 1 Carbs: 20 Fiber: 2 Protein: 5

NOVEMBER 26: THE LOTUS CRUISE

Serves 1

This Far East–flavored spiced smoothie is addictive! Full of fiber, probiotics and warming spices, this combo is a great daily digestive.

Ingredients:

1 Medjool date

½ cup rice milk

½ cup nonfat Greek yogurt

¼ teaspoon cardamom

1 pinch of cinnamon

Directions:

Combine all ingredients in a high-power blender or food processor and blend until smooth.

Drink immediately.

> **CULINARY TIP** *Dates and prunes both add sweetness to smoothies but have slightly different flavors. Keep your favorite dried fruit on hand to use for sweetening smoothies.*

Nutrition Facts (per serving):
Calories: 193 Fat: 1 Carbs: 34 Fiber: 2 Protein: 13

POMEGRANATE JUICE SMOOTHIES

NOVEMBER 27: DETOX SMOOTHIE

Serves 2

This juicy, fresh smoothie is a vehicle for detoxifying supplements that help maintain a healthy metabolism. Hemp provides a rich array of minerals, including zinc, calcium, phosphorous, magnesium and iron. Adding soluble fiber to a smoothie helps reduce the overall glycemic load.

Ingredients:

1 cup frozen wild blueberries

½ cup pomegranate juice

½ cup ice

2 tablespoons hulled hemp seed

1 teaspoon fiber supplement

½ teaspoon probiotic supplement

Directions:

Combine all ingredients in a high-power blender or food processor and blend until smooth. Drink immediately.

Nutrition Facts (per serving):
Calories: 119 Fat: 3 Carbs: 20 Fiber: 5 Protein: 3

NOVEMBER 28: POMEGRANATE BREEZE

Serves 2

This super antioxidant mix is sweet, with the scent of vanilla and lemon. Just 2 to 3 ounces of pomegranate juice daily reduces the oxidation process of fats in our bodies, protecting us from the accumulation of unhealthy fats in our arteries.

Ingredients:

1 cup ice

½ cup pomegranate juice

½ cup frozen wild blueberries

2 tablespoons chia seed

1 teaspoon lemon juice

1 teaspoon vanilla extract

Directions:

Combine all ingredients in a high-power blender or food processor and blend until smooth. Drink immediately.

CULINARY **TIP** *Boost the amount of vanilla and lemon if you prefer a more intense flavor.*

Nutrition Facts (per serving):
Calories: 127 Fat: 5 Carbs: 14 Fiber: 8 Protein: 3

NOVEMBER 29: COOL BLUE MORNING

Serves 2

This blend is a magic combination of flavors and nutrients, making it the perfect daily smoothie for health and hedonism.

Ingredients:

½ cup brewed green tea

½ cup frozen wild blueberries

½ cup pomegranate juice

¼ cup ice

1 tablespoon chia seed

½ teaspoon turmeric powder

Directions:

Combine all ingredients in a high-power blender or food processor and blend until smooth. Drink immediately.

CULINARY TIP *Fresh turmeric root or dried powdered turmeric can be used. Ground turmeric powder is more widely available and is easier to use in smoothies.*

Nutrition Facts (per serving):
Calories: 121 Fat: 5 Carbs: 14 Fiber: 8 Protein: 3

NOVEMBER 30: ANTIOXIDANT ICY

Serves 2

This drink is the perfect blend, as the blueberries sweeten up the astringent pomegranate. Pomegranate juice and wild blueberries are two of the richest food sources of antioxidants discovered to date.

Ingredients:

1 cup pomegranate juice

½ cup ice

½ cup frozen wild blueberries

2 tablespoons chia seed

Directions:

Combine all ingredients in a high-power blender or food processor and blend until smooth. Drink immediately.

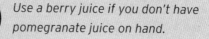

CULINARY TIP *Use a berry juice if you don't have pomegranate juice on hand.*

Nutrition Facts (per serving):
Calories: 154 Fat: 5 Carbs: 22 Fiber: 8 Protein: 3

CHAPTER 15

December Smoothies

CULTURED COCONUT MILK SMOOTHIES

DECEMBER 1: CHERRY APRÉS PLAY CAFÉ

Serves 1

This rich and replenishing smoothie is a powerhouse of potassium. The caffeine in coffee can function as a pain reliever, hence its use in over-the-counter pain medications to reduce headaches and muscle pain.

Ingredients:

½ frozen banana

½ cup cultured coconut milk

½ cup ice

½ cup frozen dark cherries

2 teaspoons instant coffee

Directions:

Combine all ingredients in a high-power blender or food processor and blend until smooth. Drink immediately.

Nutrition Facts (per serving):
Calories: 135 Fat: 3 Carbs: 29 Fiber: 5 Protein: 2

DECEMBER 2: BLUEBERRIES AND COCONUT CREAM

Serves 2

This creamy, sweet, high-energy combination is rich in protein from the yogurt and hemp seed.

Ingredients:

½ frozen banana

½ cup cultured coconut milk

½ cup coconut water

½ cup frozen blueberries

½ cup nonfat Greek yogurt

2 tablespoons hulled hemp seed

Directions:

Combine all ingredients in a high-power blender or food processor and blend until smooth. Drink immediately.

CULINARY TIP *You can use whole hulled hemp seeds or ground hemp seed protein powder in this recipe. I use Bob's Red Mill brand because it has a mild flavor and it's easy to find at my local grocery store.*

Nutrition Facts (per serving):
Calories: 150 Fat: 5 Carbs: 20 Fiber: 4 Protein: 9

DECEMBER 3: CHERRY BIOTIC BLAST

Serves 2

Indulge yourself in this creamy delight.

Ingredients:

½ frozen banana

½ cup cultured coconut milk

½ cup frozen cherries

½ cup nonfat Greek yogurt

½ cup ice

Directions:

Combine all ingredients in a high-power blender
or food processor and blend until smooth.
Drink immediately.

Nutrition Facts (per serving):
Calories: 101 Fat: 2 Carbs: 17 Fiber: 2 Protein: 7

DECEMBER 4: ATHLETE'S CHOCOLATE BREAKFAST

Serves 2

This smoothie is creamy and rich in chocolate flavor,
and the cultured coconut milk provides probiotics
that support muscle development.

Ingredients:

1 frozen banana

½ cup cultured coconut milk

½ cup ice

½ cup nonfat Greek yogurt

2 tablespoons hulled hemp seed

2 tablespoons unsweetened cocoa powder

Directions:

Combine all ingredients in a high-power blender
or food processor and blend until smooth.
Drink immediately.

CULINARY TIP *Add a pitted date or two if you'd like to sweeten this smoothie.*

Nutrition Facts (per serving):
Calories: 168 Fat: 6 Carbs: 21 Fiber: 4 Protein: 10

DECEMBER 5: CHOCOLATE-COVERED CHERRIES

Serves 1

Drink away your chocolate cravings with this tart,
sweet coconut smoothie. Unsweetened cocoa powder
is very nutritious and adds metabolism-improving
antioxidants to any smoothie. Hemp seed is a rich
source of the coveted omega-3 fatty acids that give
our hair and skin a beautiful luster.

Ingredients:

½ cup cultured coconut milk
¼ cup frozen dark cherries
¼ cup ice
1 tablespoon hulled hemp seed
½ tablespoon unsweetened cocoa powder

Directions:

Combine all ingredients in a high-power blender
or food processor and blend until smooth.
Drink immediately.

Nutrition Facts (per serving):
Calories: 114 Fat: 7 Carbs: 12 Fiber: 4 Protein: 4

DECEMBER 6: PEACHY COLADA

Serves 2

This smoothie is south of the border meets the heartland. It's a tropical treat available year round. Cultured coconut milk contains healthful probiotics just like yogurt and kefir, and it's delicious, too!

Ingredients:

1 cup cultured coconut milk

¼ cup frozen peach

¼ cup frozen mango

¼ cup unsweetened fine macaroon coconut

¼ cup ice

Directions:

Combine all ingredients in a high-power blender or food processor and blend until smooth. Drink immediately.

CULINARY TIP *Coconut water can be used in place of coconut milk, which changes the texture from one that resembles a milkshake to one that's like a sorbet.*

Nutrition Facts (per serving):
Calories: 118 Fat: 9 Carbs: 10 Fiber: 4 Protein: 1

DECEMBER 7: PURPLE PINEAPPLE

Serves 2

This energy-boosting combination is creamy, tart and tangy.

Ingredients:

1 cup cultured coconut milk

½ cup frozen blackberries

½ cup frozen pineapple

½ cup nonfat Greek yogurt

Directions:

Combine all ingredients in a high-power blender or food processor and blend until smooth. Drink immediately.

Nutrition Facts (per serving):
Calories: 113 Fat: 3 Carbs: 17 Fiber: 4 Protein: 7

DECEMBER 8: CREAMY WILD BLUEBERRY

Serves 2

This smoothie is like an old-fashioned blueberry milkshake. The cultured coconut milk provides probiotics, and the wild blueberries are one of our richest sources of polyphenols.

Ingredients:

1 cup cultured coconut milk

1 cup frozen wild blueberries

½ cup nonfat Greek yogurt

Directions:

Combine all ingredients in a high-power blender or food processor and blend until smooth. Drink immediately.

CULINARY TIP *Use any milk alternative you prefer in this smoothie. Greek yogurt gives this drink the bulk of its protein.*

Nutrition Facts (per serving):
Calories: 104 Fat: 3 Carbs: 15 Fiber: 5 Protein: 7

DECEMBER 9: VANILLA DREAM SHAKE

Serves 2

The heady vanilla bean flavor is brilliant in this creamy, cool blend. Dates provide a sweet flavor and they're rich in fiber.

Ingredients:

2 Medjool dates

½ vanilla bean

1 cup frozen wild blueberries

½ cup cultured coconut milk

½ cup nonfat Greek yogurt

Directions:

Combine all ingredients in a high-power blender or food processor and blend until smooth. Drink immediately.

CULINARY TIP *If you don't have a high-power blender, use vanilla extract instead of a vanilla bean.*

Nutrition Facts (per serving):
Calories: 152 Fat: 2 Carbs: 32 Fiber: 5 Protein: 7

DECEMBER 10: COCONUT AND MEDJOOL DATES

Serves 1

Enjoy this creamy and cool date ambrosia blend!

Ingredients:

2 Medjool dates

½ cup cultured coconut milk

½ cup nonfat Greek yogurt

¼ cup ice

Directions:

Combine all ingredients in a high-power blender or food processor and blend until smooth. Drink immediately.

CULINARY TIP *Cultured coconut milk tastes like yogurt or kefir with a tinge of tartness, which pairs well with the sweet earthy flavor of dates. "Cultured" indicates that the product contains healthful probiotics, such as lactobacillus acidophilus.*

Nutrition Facts (per serving):
Calories: 234 Fat: 3 Carbs: 44 Fiber: 5 Protein: 13

DECEMBER 11: TROPICAL POWER SMOOTHIE

Serves 2

This smoothie is light but full-bodied with coconut and cream.

Ingredients:

1 cup pineapple

½ cup cultured coconut milk

½ cup coconut water

½ cup nonfat Greek yogurt

Directions:

Combine all ingredients in a high-power blender or food processor and blend until smooth.

Drink immediately.

CULINARY TIP *Add ice if you prefer a colder, thicker drink.*

Nutrition Facts (per serving):
Calories: 102 Fat: 2 Carbs: 17 Fiber: 2 Protein: 7

GREEK YOGURT SMOOTHIES

DECEMBER 12: TART RASPBERRY VANILLA

Serves 2

Vanilla beans provide intense flavor to this creamy berry smoothie. Vanilla also provides high levels of antioxidants, which help eliminate free radicals that damage our skin, aging it prematurely.

Ingredients:

½ vanilla bean

½ cup coconut water

½ cup frozen raspberries

½ cup nonfat Greek yogurt

½ cup ice

1 teaspoon lemon juice

Directions:

Combine all ingredients in a high-power blender or food processor and blend until smooth.

Drink immediately.

CULINARY TIP *Vanilla beans can be expensive, but when purchased from bulk bins, they're surprisingly affordable because they don't weigh much.*

Nutrition Facts (per serving):
Calories: 59 Fat: 0 Carbs: 9 Fiber: 2 Protein: 6

DECEMBER 13: VANILLA PROTEIN POWER

Serves 2

This is a delicious vanilla and banana blend that is so good, you may want it every day!

Ingredients:

½ frozen banana

½ cup coconut water

½ cup nonfat Greek yogurt

½ cup ice

1 teaspoon vanilla extract

Directions:

Combine all ingredients in a high-power blender or food processor and blend until smooth. Drink immediately.

Nutrition Facts (per serving):
Calories: 76 Fat: 0 Carbs: 12 Fiber: 1 Protein: 6

DECEMBER 14: HARD BODY FUEL

Serves 2

This smoothie is creamy with almond nibbles and layers of spices and flavors.

Ingredients:

½ frozen banana

½ cup coconut water

½ cup nonfat Greek yogurt

¼ cup roasted and chopped almonds

¼ teaspoon turmeric powder

1 pinch of ground cardamom

1 pinch of fresh ground black pepper

Directions:

Combine all ingredients in a high-power blender
or food processor and blend until smooth.
Drink immediately.

CULINARY TIP *Coconut water contains cytokine, a plant-growth hormone that regulates cell division and reduces skin wrinkles over time.*

Nutrition Facts (per serving):
Calories: 230 Fat: 14 Carbs: 16 Fiber: 5 Protein: 12

DECEMBER 15: DARK CHOCOLATE BANANA

Serves 2

This creamy smoothie has a rich and bitter cocoa
flavor. The cocoa contains the flavonol epicatechin
that helps our bodies burn calories rather than storing
them away as body fat.

Ingredients:

1 frozen banana

1 cup oat milk

½ cup nonfat Greek yogurt

2 tablespoons unsweetened cocoa powder

Directions:

Combine all ingredients in a high-power blender
or food processor and blend until smooth.
Drink immediately.

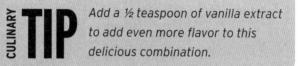

CULINARY TIP *Add a ½ teaspoon of vanilla extract to add even more flavor to this delicious combination.*

Nutrition Facts (per serving):
Calories: 171 Fat: 2 Carbs: 30 Fiber: 4 Protein: 10

DECEMBER 16: TART CHERRY CREAM

Serves 2

Creamy, pink and sweet, this is a classic comfort food
smoothie! The tart cherries used in this recipe contain
anthocyanins and proanthocyanidins that help reduce
inflammation, thus reducing water weight.

Ingredients:

1 cup hemp milk

1 cup frozen tart cherries

½ cup nonfat Greek yogurt

1 teaspoon vanilla extract

Directions:

Combine all ingredients in a high-power blender
or food processor and blend until smooth.
Drink immediately.

CULINARY TIP *Frozen cherries have had their pits already removed and give smoothies a frosty texture.*

Nutrition Facts (per serving):
Calories: 145 Fat: 3 Carbs: 21 Fiber: 2 Protein: 8

DECEMBER 17: CREAMY COCONUT

Serves 2

Coconut and banana are a perfect combination in this smoothie, with an edge of chocolate and peanut butter.

Ingredients:

1 Medjool date

½ frozen banana

½ cup coconut water

½ cup nonfat Greek yogurt

1 tablespoon unsweetened cocoa powder

1 tablespoon peanut butter

Directions:

Combine all ingredients in a high-power blender or food processor and blend until smooth.
Drink immediately.

Nutrition Facts (per serving):
Calories: 160 Fat: 4 Carbs: 23 Fiber: 3 Protein: 9

DECEMBER 18: COFFEE ALMOND CREAM

Serves 2

This roasted almond cream treat has aromatic layers of coffee and cocoa. The healthful fats from the nuts and yogurt provide energizing amino acids for hours of nutritious fuel. For those who want to gain muscle weight, a smoothie of 250-350 calories after a workout will support muscle development and boost blood sugar to help support energy levels in the hours after exertion.

Ingredients:

½ frozen banana

½ cup coconut water

½ cup roasted and chopped almonds

½ cup nonfat Greek yogurt

1 teaspoon instant coffee

1 teaspoon unsweetened cocoa powder

Directions:

Combine all ingredients in a high-power blender
or food processor and blend until smooth.
Drink immediately.

CULINARY TIP Fresh brewed coffee can be used
in place of instant coffee. Use a
¼ cup of brewed coffee to replace
1 teaspoon of instant coffee.

Nutrition Facts (per serving):
Calories: 255 Fat: 17 Carbs: 20 Fiber: 5 Protein: 8

DECEMBER 19: MEDITERRANEAN MORNING

Serves 2

This smoothie is fresh and aromatic with rich
spice flavors.

Ingredients:

1 frozen banana

½ cup coconut water

½ cup ice

½ cup nonfat Greek yogurt

1 teaspoon coconut nectar

1 pinch of ground cinnamon

1 pinch of fresh ground nutmeg

Directions:

Combine all ingredients in a high-power blender
or food processor and blend until smooth.
Drink immediately.

Nutrition Facts (per serving):
Calories: 96 Fat: 0 Carbs: 19 Fiber: 2 Protein: 7

DECEMBER 20: BEACH BODY FUEL

Serves 2

This protein-rich and creamy banana blend has blueberries, which contain pterostilbene and resveratrol–antioxidants that may help protect against cancer.

Ingredients:

½ frozen banana

½ cup coconut water

½ cup ice

½ cup frozen wild blueberries

½ cup nonfat Greek yogurt

2 tablespoons hulled hemp seed

Directions:

Combine all ingredients in a high-power blender or food processor and blend until smooth. Drink immediately.

Nutrition Facts (per serving):
Calories: 132 Fat: 3 Carbs: 18 Fiber: 3 Protein: 9

DECEMBER 21: THE FAT MELTER

Serves 2

The Greek yogurt in this recipe is a protein powerhouse that helps maintain muscle while shedding body fat. It also helps keep hunger in check for hours.

Ingredients:

½ frozen banana

1 cup coconut water

½ cup nonfat Greek yogurt

½ cup ice

2 tablespoons unsweetened cocoa powder

½ teaspoon turmeric powder

Directions:

Combine all ingredients in a high-power blender or food processor and blend until smooth. Drink immediately.

Nutrition Facts (per serving):
Calories: 101 Fat: 1 Carbs: 17 Fiber: 2 Protein: 7

DECEMBER 22: SKINNY ELIXIR

Serves 2

Drink-up to slim-down with this creamy and spicy smoothie designed to melt away water weight. Hemp seed provides omega-3 fatty acids that improve leptin signaling in the brain, which increases fat burning and decreases hunger signals.

Ingredients:

1 frozen banana

½ cup coconut water

½ cup nonfat Greek yogurt

1 tablespoon hulled hemp seed

½ teaspoon vanilla extract

½ teaspoon turmeric powder

Directions:

Combine all ingredients in a high-power blender
or food processor and blend until smooth.
Drink immediately.

Nutrition Facts (per serving):
Calories: 122 Fat: 2 Carbs: 19 Fiber: 2 Protein: 8

FRESH MANGO SMOOTHIES

DECEMBER 23: CHERRY MANGO FREEZE

Serves 2

This mango smoothie is sweet and cool with a little
turmeric flavor.

Ingredients:

1 cup coconut water

½ cup frozen cherries

½ cup mango

2 tablespoons chia seed

½ teaspoon turmeric powder

Directions:

Combine all ingredients in a high-power blender
or food processor and blend until smooth.
Drink immediately.

Nutrition Facts (per serving):
Calories: 140 Fat: 5 Carbs: 19 Fiber: 7 Protein: 4

DECEMBER 24: VANILLA MANGO

Serves 2

Watermelon juiciness combines beautifully with the exotic mango in this vanilla-scented and lightly sweet smoothie.

Ingredients:

1 cup watermelon

1 cup mango

2 tablespoons chia seed

½ teaspoon vanilla extract

Directions:

Combine all ingredients in a high-power blender or food processor and blend until smooth. Drink immediately.

Nutrition Facts (per serving):
Calories: 145 Fat: 5 Carbs: 19 Fiber: 8 Protein: 4

DECEMBER 25: VANILLA MANGO DREAM

Serves 2

This perfect, simple blend uses vanilla extract, which has been found to reduce nausea.

Ingredients:

½ frozen banana

½ cup mango

½ cup ice

½ cup coconut water

2 tablespoons chia seed

1 teaspoon vanilla extract

Directions:
Combine all ingredients in a high-power blender
or food processor and blend until smooth.
Drink immediately.

Nutrition Facts (per serving):
Calories: 137 Fat: 5 Carbs: 17 Fiber: 7 Protein: 4

DECEMBER 26: MANGO CHERRY CREAM

Serves 2

The sweet, tropical mango flavor is emphasized in
this creamy blend.

Ingredients:
½ frozen banana
½ cup mango
½ cup unfiltered apple juice
½ cup frozen cherries
½ cup nonfat Greek yogurt

Directions:
Combine all ingredients in a high-power blender
or food processor and blend until smooth.
Drink immediately.

Nutrition Facts (per serving):
Calories: 136 Fat: 0 Carbs: 28 Fiber: 2 Protein: 7

DECEMBER 27: MANGO CHERRY

Serves 2

Tart mango with sweet cherries is a perfect flavor combination in this smoothie.

Ingredients:

½ frozen banana

½ cup mango

½ cup unfiltered apple juice

½ cup frozen sweet cherries

½ cup ice

2 tablespoons chia seed

Directions:

Combine all ingredients in a high-power blender or food processor and blend until smooth. Drink immediately.

Nutrition Facts (per serving):
Calories: 173 Fat: 5 Carbs: 27 Fiber: 8 Protein: 4

DECEMBER 28: MELLOW MANGO

Serves 2

This light and frosty mango blend is simple and not too sweet.

Ingredients:

1 cup brewed green tea

1 cup mango

½ cup ice

2 tablespoons hulled hemp seed

Directions:

Combine all ingredients in a high-power blender or food processor and blend until smooth. Drink immediately.

CULINARY TIP *If you like the flavor of hemp seed, increase the amount by 1 additional tablespoon, and it will up* the protein content of this drink.

Nutrition Facts (per serving):
Calories: 94 Fat: 3 Carbs: 14 Fiber: 2 Protein: 3

DECEMBER 29: COOL TROPICAL BREEZE

Serves 2

This refreshing drink has full-bodied tropical flavors, with tart mango and bright citrus. Mangoes have magneferin and lactase enzymes, which support digestion.

Ingredients:

½ frozen banana

½ cup coconut water

½ cup mango

½ cup ice

2 tablespoons chia seed

1 tablespoon lime juice

Directions:

Combine all ingredients in a high-power blender or food processor and blend until smooth. Drink immediately.

CULINARY TIP *If you use frozen mango rather than fresh, it will thicken up the texture of this smoothie.*

Nutrition Facts (per serving):
Calories: 131 Fat: 5 Carbs: 17 Fiber: 7 Protein: 4

DECEMBER 30: MANGO AVOCADO LIME

Serves 2

This recipe is a tropical blend of fruit and coconut flavors. Avocados contain healthful monounsaturated fatty acids, which reduce appetite and help keep blood sugar steady.

Ingredients:

½ frozen banana

¼ avocado

1 cup fresh mango

½ cup frozen wild blueberries

2 tablespoons chia seed

1 teaspoon lime juice

½ teaspoon coconut extract

Directions:

Combine all ingredients in a high-power blender or food processor and blend until smooth.

Drink immediately.

Nutrition Facts (per serving):
Calories: 197 Fat: 8 Carbs: 27 Fiber: 11 Protein: 5

POMEGRANATE JUICE SMOOTHIE

DECEMBER 31: SKINNY BERRY POM

Serves 2

This smoothie has weight-loss nutrients galore and is bursting with flavor! Whey protein powders are rich in high-quality and easy-to-digest protein.

Ingredients:

1 cup frozen wild blueberries

½ cup pomegranate juice

½ cup ice

2 tablespoons chia seed

2 tablespoons vanilla-flavored protein powder

Directions:

Combine all ingredients in a high-power blender or food processor and blend until smooth. Drink immediately.

CULINARY TIP *The vanilla-flavored protein powder is sweet enough to take the bitter edge off the pomegranate juice.*

Nutrition Facts (per serving):
Calories: 161 Fat: 5 Carbs: 20 Fiber: 9 Protein: 7

ACKNOWLEDGMENTS

I am grateful for the following contributions by colleagues and friends in creating *365 Skinny Smoothies*.

First and foremost, I offer my gratitude to my kind and wise editors, Sarah Pelz and Becca Hunt, who were able to turn a manuscript that was heavy in medical nutrition jargon into a user-friendly, weight-loss tool.

Natasha Graf for her exceptional editing skills and attention to detail.

The ever-positive and always helpful Helen Gray, aka "Helpful Helen," for her many hours of high-speed and accurate nutrition analysis.

Linda Landkammer and Robin Nye, my taste-test team, for all of their feedback that helped me perfect these recipes.

Matias Booth for his hot and spicy recipe concepts.

Max Grover, my "smoothie muse," for his enthusiasm, supply runs to the grocery store and creative combinations influenced by his travels in San Miguel de Allende.

I also appreciate the generous contributions from companies and organizations that supplied high-quality tools and healthy products: Epicurean cutting boards and utensils, Shun knives, MacGourmet Nutrition analysis software, Sunpentown SPT blenders, Hamilton Beach blenders, Tribest blenders, Blendtec blenders, Calphalon, Northwest Wild Foods berries, Bob's Red Mill coconut and hemp seed, Pacific Foods milks, Wild Blueberry Association of North America and the blueberry farmers Jasper Wyman & Son (aka Wyman's of Maine), FAGE nonfat Greek yogurt, Green Valley Organics yogurt, Nature Factor organic coconut water and Zico coconut water.

I also want to extend my gratitude to Up Country Bakery Cafe in Captain Cook and Kona on The Big Island of Hawaii for their inspirational smoothie ideas sent by Antoinette Sharfin.

GLOSSARY OF TERMS

Aflatoxin: Aflatoxins are common, toxic fungi that grow on peanuts and a trigger of peanut allergies.

Anthocyanins: Anthocyanins are colorful flavonoid nutrients that have potential health effects against cancer, aging, inflammation, diabetes and bacterial infections.

Antioxidant: An antioxidant is a molecule that inhibits the oxidation of other molecules, which may provide protection against dementia, diabetes, rheumatoid arthritis and heart disease.

Aseptic packaging: Tetra Pak is the maker of the aseptic packaging used for milk alternatives. Their contents do not need to be refrigerated until the package is opened, which gives them a long shelf life.

Bioflavonoids: (See the entry for "Flavonoids.")

Blood sugar: The level of sugar in the bloodstream indicates how effectively our bodies are using sugar from the food we eat to create energy. Blood sugar testing is a common and simple test that those with diabetes use to determine whether they need to eat or take insulin.

Cultivated: Cultivated refers to foods that are agriculturally grown for consumption. For example, most blueberries are cultivated and grown on farms, whereas wild blueberries are collected from bushes growing in their natural environment.

Diabetes: Diabetes mellitus, or diabetes, is a disorder of the metabolism in which the pancreas isn't making enough insulin or the cells don't respond to the insulin that is produced resulting in high blood sugar levels (hyperglycemia).

Electrolytes: Electrolytes are minerals such as sodium,

potassium, calcium, magnesium, chloride and phosphate that control electrical conduction and hydration in our bodies. Fruits, fruit juices and coconut water are excellent natural sources of these minerals.

Ellagic acid: Ellagic acid is a natural antioxidant found in many fruits and vegetables, such as blackberries, cranberries, pomegranate, raspberries, strawberries, grapes and peaches.

Ellagitannins: Ellagitannins are natural antioxidants that provide vitamin C, vitamin K and free radical–scavenging polyphenols.

Flavonoids: Bioflavonoids, or flavonoids, are plant pigments such as quercetin, which occur naturally in onions and citrus fruit. They play a role in cancer protection and help strengthen blood vessels, thus reducing risk for aneurisms, bruising and varicose veins.

Flavonols: Flavonols are a class of flavanoids found in many fruits and vegetables. They include quercetin and kaempferol, which play an important role in our liver function and in the detoxification of enviromental toxins and medications.

Folate: Folate is a B vitamin (aka B_9) that plays a primary role in cell division and is naturally occurring in foods such as leafy greens, sunflower seeds, orange juice, pineapple juice, cantaloupe, honeydew melon, grapefruit juice, bananas, raspberries, strawberries and tomato juice. We need to take in about 400 mcg per day to avoid deficiency.

Free radical: A free radical is an atom, molecule or ion that is highly reactive, meaning it can cause damaging reactions to occur in the body. Antioxidants are the nutrients that bond to them, rendering them inactive and harmless.

Genetically modified organisms (GMOs): Fruits, vegetables, dairy and now even meats have been manipulated by chemical corporations in a process called genetic modification. The actual genetic material of these foods have been altered. They should be avoided when possible, as they carry health risks such as higher chemical residue and food reactions (allergies). Foods that are labeled organic are a healthier choice as they are non-GMO.

Glycemic load: The glycemic load of food is a number that estimates how much the food will raise a person's blood sugar after eating or drinking it. The glycemic load is determined based on the food's Glycemic Index minus its fiber load.

Glycogen: Glycogen is the storage of sugar as bundles of glucose in muscle and the liver, where our bodies access it when needed (such as when we strenuously exercise or in times of starvation).

Hormones: Hormones are the chemical messengers that regulate our endocrine systems.

Hydration: Hydration levels indicate how much water is in our bodies and how well we are able to absorb and maintain water levels. When we are low in water, we can become dehydrated, which can cause physical symptoms, such as headaches, false-hunger signals, joint pain and backaches.

Hypoglycemia: Hypo (low) and glycemia (blood sugar) is the term used for an imbalance in blood sugar that can cause symptoms such as weakness, fatigue and brain fog. When we have low blood sugar, we need to eat or drink carbohydrates to raise our blood sugar to a healthy level.

Inflammation: Inflammation or inflamed tissues can cause swelling, edema, redness and heat. It can also cause puffiness, distended stomach and puckering in the thighs, which we often think of as cellulite.

Insulin: Insulin is the hormone made by the pancreas that pulls sugar into cells to be used as energy from the bloodstream. Those who are insulin dependent take insulin injections to manage their blood sugar levels.

Lipolysis: Lipolysis is the breakdown of lipids (fat) for the body to use as energy.

Melatonin: Melatonin is the hormone that regulates sleep (circadian rhythms) and is an antioxidant that protects our cells from genetic damage.

Metabolism: Metabolism generally refers to the digestion of foods and their transport throughout the body.

Metabolic syndrome: Metabolic syndrome is the term used for a group of disorders, such as obesity and insulin resistance, that increase the risk for heart disease and diabetes.

Nectar: Fruit nectars, such as mango, papaya, and blueberry, are richer, sweeter and thicker than most fruit juices. They are unstrained and contain more pulp.

Noradrenaline: Noradrenaline is a hormone and a neurotransmitter that controls many biological functions, including our focus, fight-or-flight response and heart rate.

Oleanolic acid: This naturally occurring triterpenoid is found in plants such as garlic and holy basil, which provides protection of the liver and immune system, reduces cancer risk and provides protection from viruses.

Pancreatic beta cells: The cells of the pancreas that produce the hormone insulin are the beta cells, which are more commonly known as the islets and Langerhans. Insulin grabs up sugar in the bloodstream and carries it into the cells, where it can be used as energy or stored as body fat.

Phytosterols: Phytosterols are naturally occurring cholesterol-lowering plant compounds found in nuts, vegetables, fruits and berries.

Polyphenols: Polyphenols are naturally occurring substances found in grape and berry skins, grape seeds, cinnamon bark, pomegranate seeds, cloves, tea leaves, red wine, coffee, chocolate, olives and extra virgin olive oil. Olives and olive oil from Spain have the highest-concentration of these health-promoting nutrients. When these nutrients are modified by intestinal microflora enzymes they provide benefits such as reducing inflammation and protecting our cells from cancer.

Probiotics: Probiotics are live, health-promoting bacteria taken as supplements or in foods such as yogurt and fermented food products, such as kimchi and sauerkraut. These bacteria are necessary for proper digestion and help us to balance our hormones; absorb nutrients; and protect us from unhealthy bacteria, viruses and fungus.

Rosmarinic acid: Rosmarinic acid is a naturally occurring phenol antioxidant found in herbs such as rosemary, oregano, sage, thyme and peppermint. It has antiviral, antibacterial, anti-inflammatory and antioxidant properties.

Tannic: Tannins often have a tannic flavor, which is astringent or slightly bitter.

Thiamine: Vitamin B_1 is also know as thiamine. This B vitamin is needed for building neurotransmitters, eyesight and proper functioning of our cardiovascular system. If we become deficient in this nutrient, we may experience symptoms such as malaise, weight loss, irritability and confusion.

Tryptophan: Tryptophan is an essential amino acid necessary for the production of serotonin, melatonin and niacin.

Ursolic acid: Ursolic acid is a strong anti-cancer agent that is naturally occurring in apples, basil, bilberries, cranberries, peppermint, rosemary, oregano, thyme and prunes.

For a complete list of references and resources used for this book, please visit **www.daniellachace.com**.

INDEX

A

B

C

G

H

I

K

L

M

R

S

T

X

Y